D0224630

COGNITIVE DECLINE

Strategies for Prevention

Pacific
WITHDRAWN
University

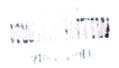

COGNITIVE DECLINE
Strategies for Prevention

Edited by

HM Fillit and RN Butler

CAMBRIDGE
UNIVERSITY PRESS

PACIFIC UNIVERSITY
LIBRARY

CAMBRIDGE UNIVERSITY PRESS
Cambridge, New York, Melbourne, Madrid, Cape Town, Singapore, São Paulo

Cambridge University Press
The Edinburgh Building, Cambridge CB2 2RU, UK

Published in the United States of America by Cambridge University Press, New York

www.cambridge.org
Information on this title: www.cambridge.org/9780521026703

© 1997 Greenwich Medical Media Ltd

This publication is in copyright. Subject to statutory exception
and to the provisions of relevant collective licensing agreements,
no reproduction of any part may take place without
the written permission of Cambridge University Press.

First published 1997
Digitally printed first paperback version by Cambridge University Press 2006

A catalogue record for this publication is available from the British Library

ISBN-13 978-0-521-02670-3 paperback
ISBN-10 0-521-02670-9 paperback

The publisher makes no representation, express or implied, with regard to the accuracy
of the information contained in this publication and cannot accept any legal responsibility or
liability for any errors or omissions that may be made.

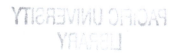
PACIFIC UNIVERSITY
LIBRARY

CONTENTS

PREFACE

When modern gerontology was born, the dementias and other forms of cognitive decline were generally considered to be inevitable and natural accompaniments of aging that were unpreventable and untreatable. Previously, mental deteriorations of old age were written off as 'senile psychosis' or 'psychosis with cerebral arteriosclerosis'. Now the dementias have become important and growing topics of productive research. We know infinitely more about central nervous system organization in general and at the molecular level in particular. Vascular dementia in various forms and Alzheimer's dementia (also likely to be in many forms) are now recognized as diseases worthy of research and, therefore, ultimately preventable and treatable. The vascular form of dementia, in particular, can already be prevented to some degree through the control of hypertension.

This book brings together investigators involved in cutting-edge research that may yield new strategies for delaying cognitive decline. It provides a useful summary of present knowledge and should stimulate further research. In addition, it should encourage primary care and specialty physicians to apply what we already know about preventing and delaying dementia in their everyday clinical practice.

There are few diseases that people fear more than the dementias. They evoke the depressing image of growing old, losing one's mind, and being sentenced to spending one's final years in indignity. Action now to build an overall research and practice strategy to prevent and delay cognitive decline in old age would reduce fears of growing old and becoming demented, as well as save billions of dollars in health care and other related costs. This would give all of us hope for a better quality of life in old age.

Howard M Fillit
Robert N Butler

ACKNOWLEDGEMENTS

The Strategies to Prevent Cognitive Decline in Late Life symposium was sponsored by The International Longevity Center (ILC-US) in the Henry L Schwartz Department of Geriatrics and Adult Development, The Mount Sinai Medical Center, New York, NY, USA.

We gratefully wish to thank the following organizations: The Henry L Schwartz Department of Geriatrics and Adult Development, Mount Sinai Medical Center; the Jewish Home and Hospital for the Aged; The Page and William Black Post-Graduate School of Medicine of the Mount Sinai School of Medicine (CUNY); The Hunter/Mount Sinai Geriatric Education Center; and the Alliance for Aging Research.

We are also grateful to the following corporations whose generosity and support were essential to the success of the symposium; Warner-Lambert Company; Merrill-Lynch and Co, Inc.; and the Geron Corporation.

We would also like to thank the following for their administrative and editorial support; Mary Bill, Financial and Budget Manager; Mia Oberlink, Communications Director, ILC-US; and Orie Costanza, Administrative Coordinator, ILC-US.

Finally, we thank NYLCare Health Plans, Inc., for their support of our effots to bring this text to publication.

Robert N Butler
Howard M Fillit

CONTRIBUTORS

RN Butler MD
BROOKDALE PROFESSOR OF GERIATRICS
AND ADULT DEVELOPMENT
and
DIRECTOR OF THE INTERNATIONAL
LONGEVITY CENTRE
The Mount Sinai Medical Center.New York

RTF Cheung

*Department of Clinical Neurological Sciences,
University of Western Ontario, London, Ontario,
Canada.*

HM Fillit MD
CORPORATE MEDICAL DIRECTOR
FOR MEDICARE
NYLCare Health Plans, New York, NY
and
CLINICAL PROFESSOR OF GERIATRICS
ANDADULT DEVELOPMENT
*The Henry L Schwartz Department of Geriatrics
and Adult Development, The Mount Sinai Medical
Center, New York, NY*

DJ Foley MS

*Epidemiology, Demography and Biometry Program,
National Institues of Health, Bethesda, Maryland*

VC Hachinski MD FRCPC DSc(MED)
CHIEF

*Department of Clinical Neurological Sciences,
University of Western Ontario, London, Ontario,
Canada*

RJ Havlik MD MPH

*Epidemiology, Demography and Biometry Program,
National Institues of Health, Bethesda, Maryland*

SK Inouye MD PhD
ASSOCIATE PROFESSOR OF MEDICINE

*Department of Internal Medicine, Yale Unicersity
School of Medicine, New Haven, CT*

R Katzman MD
PROFESSOR OF NEUROSCIENCES
University of California, San Diego USA

BS McEwen PhD
PROFESSOR AND HEAD
NEUROENDOCRINOLOGY

*Harold and Margaret Milliken Laboratory of
Neuroendocrinology Rockerfeller Universiy,
New York*

E Simonsick
EPIDEMIOLOGIST

*Epidemiology, Demography and Biometry Program,
NIA, NIH, Bethesda*

K Warner Schaie
EVAN PUGH PROFESSOR OF HUMAN
DEVELOPMENT AND PSYCHOLOGY
and
DIRECTOR OF GERONTOLOGY CENTRE

The Pennsylvania State University

LR White MD MPH
CHIEF
*Asia-Pacific Office, Honolulu-Asia Aging Study,
Honolulu, Hawaii*

SL Willis
PROFESSOR OF HUMAN DEVELOPMENT

Pennsylvania State University

1

THE CLINICAL SIGNIFICANCE
OF NORMAL COGNITIVE DECLINE
IN LATE LIFE

Howard Fillit

The nature and extent of changes in cognitive function associated with aging have been long investigated and are now reasonably well defined.[1-3] By the age of 70, most people have a significant, but manageable, decline in some cognitive abilities compared to their mid-life, including some deterioration in memory performance, speed of cognitive processing, and executive functions. In contrast, vocabulary and knowledge continue to grow with aging. As a result of changes in cognitive ability, older individuals may develop coping strategies which focus on their strengths in order to maximize function and compensate for the loss of abilities in specific areas.[4]

In recognition of changes in cognitive function with aging reported by older individuals as clinically significant, the term 'benign sensescent forgetfulness' was introduced.[5] This term attempted to distinguish a syndrome of cognitive impairment in elderly people who complained of memory impairment, but were not demented. It served a useful purpose for clinicians and patients because it recognized (rather than denied) the fact that elderly people frequently are aware of and complain of cognitive difficulties which initiate health seeking behaviors for effective means of management or treatment. The term also distinguished individuals without such complaints who presumably either do not suffer cognitive decline with aging or are unaware or not troubled by these changes.

Subsequently, the National Institute of Mental Health recognized and addressed the issue of clinically significant cognitive decline associated with aging which does not meet criteria for dementia by establishing a diagnosis of age-associated memory impairment'.[6] Generally, the criteria for this diagnosis include subjective complaints of memory loss associated with objective measures of memory impairment but otherwise perserved global intellectual function in a person over the age of 50 years. Most recently, the term 'age-related cognitive decline' was incorporated into the

DSM-IV,[7] while the International Psychogeriatrics Association created the term 'aging-associated cognitive decline',[8] providing increasing clinical recognition of the problem of cognitive decline with apparently normal aging, and further attempting to define and refine the diagnosis. Recent reviews have also discussed the complex relationship between cognitive aging, age-associated memory impairment and Alzheimer's disease.[9]

As in other organ systems, cognitive decline may not be an inevitable or irreversible component of normal aging. Longitudinal studies have been conducted to investigate normal cognitive aging.[3] Factors which are associated with robust cognitive health in late life include:

- Avoidance of cardiovascular and other chronic diseases.
- A favorable environment (high socioeconomic status).
- Involvement in a stimulating environment.
- A flexible personality in middle age.
- Marriage to a spouse with high cognitive status.
- Maintenance of high levels of perceptual processing speed.
- High satisfaction with life accomplishments.
- Maintenance of vision and hearing.

In contrast to age-associated cognitive decline, a diagnosis of dementia is made when cognitive impairment is greater than that found with normal aging, affects two or more cognitive domains, and affects the person's ability to function.[10,11] Dementia is characterized by loss of memory, language, the ability to perform complex tasks (such as feeding and dressing) and other cognitive abilities. Dementia is also often associated with a change in personality and mood disorders, including depression and agitation. Much research has been directed towards understanding the causes of the dementia, particularly Alzheimer's disease and vascular causes. Vascular factors, particularly hypertension and stroke, probably play a role in about half of all cases of dementia (including vascular dementias and the mixed dementias), and vascular-related dementias may be the most common type of dementia in the very old.[12-14] Dementia may affect up to 25% of individuals over the age of 80 and for society is an enormous financial and social burden.[15]

Few studies have extensively investigated the clinical relationship between age-associated cognitive impairment and dementia.[9,16,17] We may generally conclude from these studies that while the majority of individuals with age-associated cognitive decline do not go on to develop dementia, a small minority of aged individuals with apparent age-associated cognitive impairment do develop progressive cognitive failure and dementia.[9,16,18] In one prospective study,[8] 59.1% of subjects met critieria for age-associated memory impairment, representing a substantial percentage of individuals in a relatively young (to a geriatrician) population with a mean age of 71.7 years. Only 9.1% of individuals with age-associated memory impairment developed dementia (primarily Alzheimer's disease) in a 3.6 year follow-up period. Those individuals who developed dementia had lower baseline scores on mental status testing compared to those subjects who did not subsequently develop dementia. Attempts have been made to identify neuropsychologic, neuroimaging and other markers which may distinguish individuals who are at risk for subsequent dementia versus those whose cognitive impairments will remain stable and within the 'normative' range.[1,19,20]

However, whether there is an etiological and/or clinical relationship between age-associated cognitive decline and dementia at all, and if so, whether this relationship is continuous or not, remains an important unanswered question[21] that has been long debated.[22,23] An etiological perspective may support the hypothesis that age-associated cognitive decline and dementia represent a continuum.[24,25] Pathologic variables associated with cognitive decline, such as amyloid deposition, neurofibrillary tangles and angiopathy are employed as relatively continuous rather than discontinuous variables in distinguishing normal brain aging from dementia.[7,26] In addition, certain common factors may contribute to both age-associated cognitive decline and to the pathogenesis of some forms of dementia. For example, hypertension may contribute to age-associated cognitive decline[27-29] and cause vascular-related dementias.[13,14,30] High levels of education and occupational achievement are also associated with both robust cognitive health[3] and a decreased incidence of dementia.[31,32] The mechanisms by which education and demanding occupations may protect against cognitive decline are poorly understood.[33] In a given individual, mild cognitive decline may represent more rapid 'aging', may be a marker for underlying disease, or may be a precursor of the early onset of dementia.

Although some degree of age-associated cognitive impairment may be practically universal among people over the age of 80,[34] the subtle effects of age-associated cognitive impairment on the older person's ability to function, quality of life and health care utilization are only beginning to be understood. Cognitive decline can clearly affect the older person's ability to function.[35-37] Problems with memory and cognitive speed of processing may create uncertainty and insecurities. Mild cognitive decline may impair quality of life by causing difficulties in social situations, driving and other instrumental or occupational activities of daily living which may ultimately contribute to loss of functional independence, limitations in community activities and other social and mental activities which could promote mental health. Cognitive impairment can also affect the quality of life and the mood of spouses.[38,39]

Cognitive impairment also may have a major impact on health care utilization,[40] contributing to medication noncompliance and a failure to make proper and timely judgements about health. Cognitive impairment clearly affects hospital utilization and hospital length of stay,[41-44] and institutionalization.[45] Mild cognitive impairment may also be predictive of subsequent mortality.[46-48] In the very old, mild cognitive impairment equivalent to age-associated memory impairment has been associated with increased mortality.[49]

The cause of age-associated cognitive decline is not known. Some studies suggest that age-associated cognitive impairment may be reversible.[50,51] A number of potentially reversible factors related to disease, lifestyle and other conditions may contribute to cognitive impairment in old age,[50] such as cardiovascular/cerebrovascular disease, hypertension,[29] episodes of delirium (acute confusional state) during an acute illness or hospitalization,[52] depression,[53] and the effects of altered metabolism of gonadal hormones[54] and steroid hormones.[55,56] Lifestyle factors,[57] including ongoing mental and physical exercise,[57-60] psychosocial stress,[61] work history and education[62] may also play a role in age-associated cognitive impairment, with some of these factors being protective against cognitive decline. The role of diet, particularly control of cholesterol and micronutrient deficiencies, and substance abuse, including smoking[30] and alcohol,[63,64] in causing cognitive impairment in old age are poorly understood.

CONCLUSION

There is now considerable scientific knowledge regarding the nature of normal cognitive decline with aging, and some of the reversible and irreversible risk factors which contribute to cognitive decline with aging. However, the clinical significance and implications for daily life of this problem are only beginning to be recognized. Although most scientific and lay interest is primarily directed to Alzheimer's disease and dementia, there is also growing public concern and awareness about cognitive aging.[65]

Robust aging is an achievable and worthwhile goal.[66] An ultimate goal of this book is to emphasize the importance of cognitive aging as a determinant of successful aging.[67] The promotion of 'robust cognitive health' in old age through preventive strategies based on an understanding of the factors that lead to cognitive decline in late life can promote the formulation of research and policy agendas which can achieve this goal in the future. The panel of experts who have contributed to this volume are all international leaders in their respective areas who are well qualified to summarize current knowledge. The synergy of their expertise provides a broad and comprehensive review of the factors leading to cognitive decline in late life.

REFERENCES

1. Dal Forno G, Kawas CH. Cognitive problems in the elderly. *Curr Opin Neurol* 1995; **8**: 256.

2. Birren JE. Age, competence, creativity and wisdom. In: Butler RN, Gleason HP (eds). Productive Aging: Enhancing Vitality in Later Life. Springer-Verlag, New York, 1985, pp 29-36.

3. Mortimer JA. Epidemiology of dementia: cross cultural comparisons. *Adv Neurol* 1990; **51**: 27.

4. Baltes PB. The aging mind: potential and limits. Gerontologist 1993; **33**: 580.

5. Kral VA. Senescent forgetfulness: benign and malignant. *Can Med Assoc J* 1962; **86**: 257.

6. Crook TH, Bartus RT, Ferris SH et al. Age associated memory impairment: proposed diagnostic criteria and measures of clinical change-report of a National Institute of Mental Health work group. *Dev Neuropsychol* 1986; **2**: 257.

7. American Psychiatric Association Committee on Nomenclature and Statistics. Diagnostic and Statistical Manual of Mental Disorders. American Psychiatric Association, Washington, DC, 1994.

8. Levy R. Aging-associated cognitive decline. *Int Psychogeriatrics* 1994; **6**: 63.

9. Reisberg B, Shulman E, Ferris SH, DeLeon MJ, Geibel V. Clinical assessments of age-associated cognitive decline and primary degenerative dementia: prognostic concomitants. *Psychopharm Bull* 1983; **19**: 734.

10. McKhann G, Drachman D, Folstein M, Katzman R, Price D, Stadlan EM. Clinical diagnosis of Alzheimer's disease: Report of the NINCDS-ADRDA work group under the auspices of the Department of Health and Human Services Task Force on Alzheimer's Disease. *Neurology* 1984; **34**:939.

11. Larson EB, Kukull WA, Katzman RL. Cognitive impairment: dementia and Alzheimer's disease. *Ann Rev Public Health* 1992; **13**: 431.

12. Larsson EB. Illnesses causing dementia in the very elderly. *N Engl J Med* 1993; **328**: 203.

13. White L. Is silent cerebrovascular disease an important cause of late-life cognitive decline? *J Am Geriatr Soc* 1996; **44**: 328.

14. Hachinski VC. Vascular dementia: a radical redefinition. *Dementia* 1994; **5**: 130.

15. Ernst RL, Hay JW. The US economic and social costs of Alzheimer's disease revisited. *Am J Pub Health* 1994; **84**: 1261.

16. Flicker C, Ferris SH, Reisberg B. Mild cognitive impairment in the elderly: predictors of dementia. *Neurology* 1991; **41**: 1006.

17. Khachaturian Z. Diagnosis of Alzheimer's disease. *Arch Neurol* 1985; **42**: 1097.

18. Hanninen T, Hallikainen M, Koivisto K et al. A followup study of age-associated memory impairment: neuropsychological predictors of dementia. *J Am Geriatr Soc* 1995; **43**: 1007.

19. Petersen RC, Smith GE, Ivnik RJ, Kokmen E, Tangalos EG. Memory function in very early Alzheimer's disease. *Neurology* 1994; **44**: 867.

20. Masur EM, Sliwinski M, Lipton RB, Blau AD, Crystal HA. Neuropsychological prediction of dementia and the absence of dementia in healthy elderly persons. *Neurology* 1994; **44**: 1427.

21. Larrabee GJ, McEntee WJ. Age-associated memory impairment: sorting out the controversies. *Neurology* 1995; **45**: 610.

22. Newton RD. The identity of Alzheimer's disease and senile dementia and their relationship to senility. *J Mental Sci* 1948; **94**: 225.

23. Neumann MA, Cohn R. Incidence of Alzheimer's disease in a large mental hospital: relation to senile psychosis and psychosis with cerebral arteriosclerosis. *AMA Arch Neurol Psychiatr* 1934; 615.

24. Von Dras DD, Blumenthal HT. Dementia of the aged: disease or atypical accelerated aging? Biopathological and psychological perspectives. *J Am Geriatr Soc* 1992; **40**: 101.

25. Brayne C, Calloway P. Normal aging, impaired cognitive function, and senile dementia of Alzheimer's type: a continuum? *Lancet* 1988; **i**: 1265.

26. Buee L, Hof PR, Bouras C et al. Pathologic alterations of the cerebral microvasculature in Alzheimer's disease and related dementing disorders. *Acta Neuropathol (Berl)* 1994; **87**: 469.

27. Hertzog C, Schaie KW, Gribbin K. Cardiovascular disease and changes in intellectual functioning from middle to old age. *J Gerontol* 1978; **33**: 872.

28. Salerno JA, Grady C, Mentis M et al. Brain metabolic function in older men with chronic essential hypertension. *J Gerontol* 1995; **50A**: M147.

29. Launer LJ, Masaki K, Petrovitch H, Foley D, Havlik RJ. The association between midlife blood pressure levels and late-life cognitive function. *JAMA* 1995; **274**: 1846.

30. Meyer JS, McClintic KI, Rogers RL, Sims P, Mortel KF. Aetiological considerations and risk factors for multi-infarct dementia. *J Neurol Neurosurg Psych* 1988; **51**: 1489.

31. Stern Y, Gurland B, Tatemichi TK, Tang MX, Wilder D, Mayeux R. Influence of education and occupation on the incidence of Alzheimer's disease. *JAMA* 1994; **271**: 1004.

32. Katzman R. Views and reviews: education and the prevalence of dementia and Alzheimer's disease. *Neurology* 1993; **43**: 13.

33. Stern Y, Alexander GE, Prohovnik I et al. Relationship between lifetime occupation and pariteal flow: implications for a reserve against Alzheimer's disease pathology. *Neurology* 1995; **45**: 55.

34. Schaie K W. The hazards of cognitive aging. *Gerontologist* 1989; **29**: 484.

35. Ensrud KE, Nevitt MC, Yunis C et al. Correlates of impaired function in older women. *J Am Geriatr Soc* 1994; **42**: 481.

36. Boult C, Kane RL, Louis TA et al. Chronic conditions that lead to functional limitation in the elderly. *J Gerontol* 1994; **49**: M28.

37. Greiner PA, Snowdon DA, Schmitt FA. The loss of independence in activities of daily living: the role of low normal cognitive function in elderly nuns. *Am J Pub Health* 1996; **86**: 62.

38. Moritz DJ, Kasl SV, Berkman LF. The health impact of living with a cognitively impaired elderly spouse: depressive symptoms and social functioning. *J Gerontol* 1986; **44**: S17.

39. Deimling GT, Bass DM. Symptoms of mental impairment among elderly adults and their effects on family caregivers. *J Gerontol* 1986; **41**: 778.

40. Ganguli M, Seaberg E, Belle S et al. Cognitive impairment and the use of health services in an elderly rural population: the MoVIES project. *J Am Geriatr Soc* 1993; **41**: 1065.

41. Binder EF, Robin LN. Cognitive impairment and length of hospital stay in older persons. *J Am Geriatr Soc* 1990; **58**: 759.

42. Fulop G, Strain JJ, Vita J, Lyons JS, Hammer JS. Impact of psychiatric comorbidity on length of hospital stay for medical/surgical patients: A preliminary report. *Am J Psych* 1987; **144**: 878.

43. Torian LV, Davidson EJ, Sell L, Fulop G, Fillit H. The effect of senile dementia on acute medical care in a geriatric medicine unit. *Int Psychogeriatr* 1992; **4**: 231.

44. Weiler PG, Lubben JE, Chi I. Cognitive impairment and hospital use. *Am J Pub Health* 1991; **81**: 1153.

45. Branch LG, Jette AM. A prospective study of long term care institutionalization among the aged. *Am J Pub Health* 1982; **72**: 1373.

46. Shapiro E, Tate RB. The impact of a mental status score and a dementia diagnosis on mortality and institutionalization. *J Aging Health* 1991; **3**: 28.

47. Liu Y, Lacroiz AZ, White LR, Kittner SJ, Wolf P. Cognitive impairment and mortality: a study of possible confounders. *Am J Epidemiol* 1990; **132**: 136.

48. Kelman HR, Thomas C, Kennedy GJ, Cheng J. Cognitive impairment and mortality in older community residents. *Am J Pub Health* 1994; **84**: 1255.

49. Johansson B, Zarit SH, Berg S. Changes in cognitive functioning of the oldest-old. *J Gerontol Psychol Sci* 1992; **47**: P75.

50. Schaie KW, Willis SL. Can decline in adult intellectual functioning be reversed? *Dev Psychol* 1986; **22**: 223.

51. Nolan KA, Blass JP. Preventing cognitive decline. *Clin Geriatr Med* 1992; **8**: 19.

52. Inouye SK. The dilemna of delirium: clinical and research controversies regarding diagnosis and evaluation of delirium in hospitalized elderly medical patients. *Am J Med* 1994; **97**: 278.

53. Blazer DG, Burchett D, Service C, George LK. The association of age and depression among the elderly: an epidemiologic exploration. *J Gerontol* 1991; **46**: M210.

54. Fillit H. Future therapeutic developments of estrogen use. *J Clin Pharmacol* 1995; **35**: s25.

55. Gould E, McEwen BS. Neuronal birth and death. *Curr Opin Neurobiol* 1993; **3**: 676.

56. McEwen BS, Coirini H, Westlind-Danielsson A *et al*. Steroid hormones as mediators of neural plasticity. *J Steroid Biochem Mol Biol* 1991; **39**: 223.

57. Emery CF, Huppert FA, Schein RL. Relationships among age, exercise, health and cognitive function in a British sample. *Gerontologist* 1995; **35**: 378.

58. Emery CF, Blumenthal JA. Effects of physical exercise on psychological and cognitive function of older adults. *Ann Behavior Med* 1991; **13**: 99.

59. Rogers RL, Meyer JS, Mortal KF. After reaching retirement age, physical activity sustains cerebral perfusion and cognition. *J Am Geriatr Soc* 1990; **38**: 123.

60. Christensen H, Mackinnon A. The association between mental, social and physical activity and cognitive performance in young and old subjects. *Age Ageing* 1993; **22**: 175.

61. Sapolsky R. Stress, the Aging Brain and the Mechanisms of Neuron Death. MIT Press, Boston, 1992.

62. Schaie KW. The course of intellectual development. Gerontologist 1994; **33**: 580.

63. Charness ME, Simon RP, Greenberg DA. Ethanol and the nervous system. *N Engl J Med* 1989; **321**: 442.

64. Lishman WA. Alcoholic dementia: a hypothesis. *Lancet* 1986; **I**: 1184.

65. Schrof JM. Brain Power. *US News and World Report* 1994; November **28**: 89 (Abstract).

66. Garfein AJ, Herzog AR. Robust aging among the young-old, old-old, and oldest-old. *J Gerontol* 1995; **50B**: S77.

67. Rowe JW, Kahn RL. Human aging: usual and successful. *Science* 1987; **237**: 143.

2

NORMAL COGNITIVE DEVELOPMENT IN ADULTHOOD

K. Warner Schaie

Cognitive psychologists have long puzzled over the paradox that although long life and its accompanying accumulation of experience ought to increase intellectual competence and wisdom we nevertheless find that for most persons advanced age brings along at least some losses in these functions. Declines in the physiological infrastructure that supports competent behavioral functioning as well as the loss of important relationships and interpersonal support systems that are common in old age, all seem to cumulatively lead to declines in levels of competence.

Our own early investigations[1] suggested that there were indeed differences in cognitive performance levels between young adults, the middle aged, and the old. But what also became clear immediately was the fact that variability among individuals within the same age range also increased markedly, and that while many older persons were at a disadvantage when compared to young adults, that this was my no means a universal phenomenon.

In trying to understand the facts of normal cognitive aging we are immediately confronted with the distinction among findings from two different types of data (cross-sectional and longitudinal) that inform our discussion. Most of the older data was cross-sectional in nature. That is, researchers compared the performance of groups of individuals that differed in age at the same point in time. By definition, these groups had grown up during different historical periods. Hence, they differed not only in age but also in their previous life experiences including important relevant factors such as attained levels of education, experience of disease, and health practices during critical periods in their development. When we observed successive population cohorts at the same ages we noted therefore that each successive generation, in young adulthood, reaches a somewhat higher cognitive performance level than does the preceding one. Given this finding, cross-sectional data will erroneously suggest substantial cognitive decline in older persons, even if individuals have remained stable throughout their life span.

Table 2.1 – Basic design of the Seattle Longitudinal Study (SLS)

Study waves					
1956	1963	1970	1977	1984	1991
S_1T_1 (N=500)	S_1T_2 (N=303)	S_1T_3 (N=162)	S_1T_4 (N=130)	S_1T_5 (N=92)	S_1T_6 (N=71)
	S_2T_2 (N=997)	S_2T_3 (N=420)	S_2T_4 (N=337)	S_2T_5 (N=204)	S_2T_6 (N=161)
		S_3T_3 (N=705)	S_3T_4 (N=340)	S_3T_5 (N=225)	S_3T_6 (N=175)
			S_4T_4 (N=612)	S_4T_5 (N=294)	S_4T_6 (N=201)
				S_5T_5 (N=628)	S_5T_6 (N=428)
					S_6T_6 (N=690)

If one wishes to understand, however, whether there is actual change within individuals as they age, one must then consider longitudinal data. These are, of course, much more difficult to obtain because the same individuals must be followed over long periods of time. One of the major problem with such studies is that progressively panel members drop out, and that one may be left primarily with the most capable survivors. Moreover, just as level of performance reached in young adulthood has changed across generations, it is also possible that the rate of aging within individuals has shifted.

There are two substantive issues that will be considered in this chapter. The first is concerned with the question as to the nature of cognitive decline in normal populations, what is its average magnitude, and how uniformly are these effects across different individuals. The second issue is concerned with the question of how static age changes in cognition might be. We ask whether there are differences across generations; for example, whether the baby boomers are going to be advantaged over today's elderly when that cohort enters old age. The second question is of particular current interest as most industrial societies are faced with the problem whether increased longevity may also mandate the extension of our work life in order to retain the viability of social security and other pension systems. Indeed, the notion of working longer makes sense only if tomorrow's aged will stay competent longer than is true today.

Some relevant data that will provide evidence for the discussion of these questions comes from a longitudinal study of adult intellectual competence, known as the Seattle Longitudinal Study, that I have conducted over the past forty years.[2, 3] This study began as my doctoral dissertation, in which I conducted a cross-sectional comparison of a random sample of 500 persons from the adult membership of one of the early health maintenance organizations over the age range from the 20s to the 70s. We have been able to follow many of these persons over long periods time, reassessing them every 7 years, and in addition have added new panels from the same HMO in order to study changes in aging patterns over successive generations. During the 40 years that this study has been progress we have assessed the intellectual functioning of over 5000 adults from young adulthood to advance old age, followed over various time periods. Table 1 shows the design of this study and the number of individuals assessed during the various data collections. Since 1989 we have also been able to study the adult offspring of many of our original study participants at comparable ages, and have therefore been able to collect data on generational differences between biologically related individuals.

FINDINGS ON NORMAL AGE CHANGES IN COGNITIVE FUNCTIONS

One of the most noteworthy findings on cognitive aging is that abilities do not change in the same manner over time as shown in longitudinal studies, nor that they show similar age differences in cross-sectional studies. If one examines cross-sectional data (see Figure 1) it appears that for many abilities there seem to be dramatic downward trends beginning with the 20s with very substantial declines as advanced old age is reached (as much as 2 SD by the 80s). However, there are important exceptions. The cross-sectional data for Verbal and Numeric abilities suggest that a peak is obtained in mid-life with relative little change in early old age, but again substantial declines as the 80s are reached.

As pointed out in the introduction, one of the reasons why we obtain such dramatic age differences in cross-sectional studies is the fact that we compare groups of different individuals who had attained different levels of performance when they were in young adulthood. Hence, when we examine comparable longitudinal data (see Figure 2), which represent changes with individuals, we note that the only ability that shows profound linear decrement from young adulthood to old age turns out to be Perceptual Speed, a direct reflection of the progressive slowing neural impulses throughout the central nervous system. An important caveat, however, requires the specification of wide individual differences, to the extent that some very old people can still make a very quick response. More important is the fact that most other abilities show gain from young adulthood into mid-life. Intellectual competence generally reaches it s peak in the 40s and 50s. This makes good sense, since most people continue to gain in experience, while the impact of a declining physiological infrastructure is not sufficiently severe to exceed the gain from experience. Nevertheless, once the 60s are reached, average declines in ability may be noted; but notice they are not as great as cross-sectional data would suggest and again they differ much across abilities.

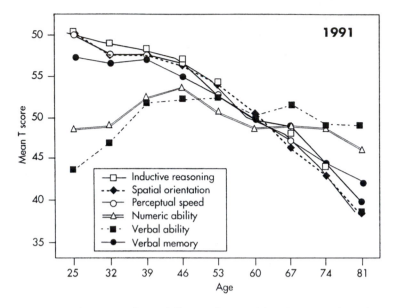

Figure 1 — *Cross-sectional age differences for six ability dimensions from the Seattle Longitudinal Study assessed in 19991.*

Source: Schaie (1994, p.307)

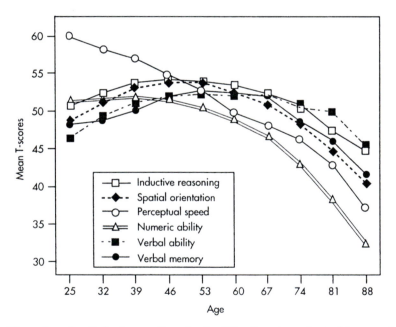

Figure 2 — *Longitudinal age gradients for six ability dimensions estimateed from cumulated within-subject age changes*

Source: Schaie (1994, p.308)

Notice that in contrast to the cross-sectional data, Numeric ability (that is the speed of making computation) declines quite dramatically with age when followed longitudinally. The cross-sectional data do not reveal this fact, because there has been a systematic decline across successive generations among Americans in their skill in manipulating numbers. Hence, even though older persons do less well than they did in their youth, they may appear as stellar performers when compared with today's high school graduates because they had developed a higher level of skill at an earlier age. By contrast, we find that Verbal ability, one that is practiced as long as we engage in any type of social interaction, actually does not peak until the 60s, and shows only very modest decline thereafter.

We need to be concerned both with the age at which decrement in abilities can be detected as well as the magnitude of the observed declines. Here I would argue that until the 60s are reached, there is very little average decline in abilities, except for the slowing in speed of performance. Hence, anyone under age 60 who is observed to be showing cognitive decline, presents us with prime signals of neuropathology; such early decline is simply not characteristic of normal aging. On the other hand it is clear that once the 80s are reached, the absence of decline would characterize a most unusual person, one who might signify for us an example of what may be possible, but certainly a representation of typical cognitive aging. With respect to differential patterns of cognitive aging, we have noted that decline is least in magnitude and occurs later on Verbal ability, while the greatest and earliest decline, on average may be observed on Perceptual Speed and Numeric ability.

What about individual differences in the occurrence of normal cognitive age changes? First of all it is clear that not all individuals decline and certainly not all individuals decline at a steady pace. As opposed to the smooth decline gradients observed in group data, individual decline seems to occur in a stair step fashion. Cognitive decline in individuals seems related typically to the occurrence of some kind of stressful event. This event may represent a drop in physiological function below an optimal threshold, or it may be an environmental impact (e.g., the loss of a support system, loss of a job, loss of a loved one). In any case, the stressful event, among other consequences, seems to result in the dropping of the cognitive behavior of the individual from a previously stable level of functioning to a lower level, at which the individual may again stabilize.

Data on the frequency of individual change over a 7-year period are presented in Figure 3 for Verbal ability and Spatial Orientation skills over three age ranges: from 60 to 67, from 67 to 74, and from 74 to 81. Notice that over these age ranges most people remain fairly stable. From 60 to 67 only about 20% of our subjects showed significant decline; of course, the proportion of persons declining rises at successive ages. But for each age group there were some persons who actually gained significantly; approximately 5% of those observed from age 74 to 81 showed such

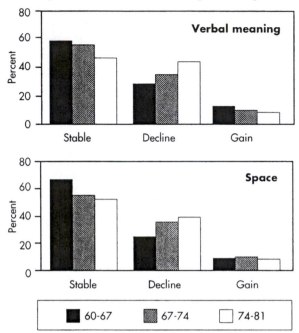

Proportions of individual change over 7 years

Figure 3 — *Proportion of individuals who significantly decline, increase or remain stable over seven years.*

Adapted from Schaie 1984

gain. What this may mean, of course, is that some persons were observed the first time when they had some disabling conditions or circumstances that could be remediated an let to a performance increase on the second test occasion (e.g., removal of a cataracts).

One might also ask whether decline occurs simultaneously across all abilities. To answer this question we have followed people over long periods of time on 5 cognitive tests: active vocabulary, spatial rotation, inductive reasoning, number additions, and word fluency. When we track people on these 5 tests, we find that by age 60, virtually all of our subjects show modest but significant decline on at least one of these tests. However, when we count the frequency of persons declining 2, 3, 4, or all 5 of these tests, we find much smaller numbers so affected. Indeed, even in the high 80s virtually none of our normal subjects have declined significantly on all 5 tests. We conclude therefore that normal cognitive aging is a highly selective phenomenon. No systematic pattern of decline can be found; individuals seem to lose ground typically on those abilities that have received relatively little exercise.[4]

FINDINGS ON GENERATIONAL DIFFERENCES

The second major issue to be addressed in this chapter is the question whether normal age changes are a stable phenomenon or whether aging occurs in different patterns and rates for successive generations. This issue obviously directly addresses our concerns with the future of aging! Generational differences in cognitive abilities have been studied in two different ways: First, we take groups in the general populations and compare their performance at the same age over successive time periods (see Willis, 1989). A second way is to compare performance within biologically related parent–offspring pairs at the same age.[5]

Findings on population cohort differences cumulated across cohorts born from 1903 to 1966 are shown in Figure 4. It appears that for some abilities there has been a systematic increase over time. This gain is particularly noteworthy for Inductive Reasoning, the ability basic to all meaningful problem solving activities, as well as for verbal memory, and to a lesser degree there has also been gain across cohorts for Spatial Orientation. But not all cohort differences in abilities are that positive. For example, Numeric ability attained a peak for those individuals who were born around 1917, and there has been a decline in numeric skills for successive cohorts ever since. In the case of the positive cohort trends, adults who have remained stable into advanced age will still be at a disadvantage when compared with the young. Conversely for Numeric ability, older adults may seem to perform remarkably well when compared to the young even though they have declined from their own peak.[2,6]

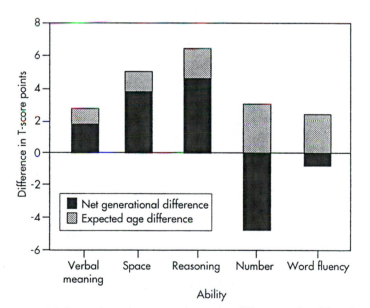

Figure 4 — PCohort gradients showing cumulative cohort differences on five abilities for cohorts born in 1907 to 1966.

Source: Schaie 1994, p 309

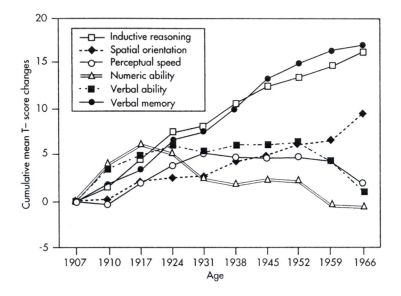

Figure 5 — *Generational differences between adult parent and offspring for the fiove abilities.*
Source: Schaie, Plomin, Willis, Gruber-Baldini, and Dutta 1992

We next asked the question whether these cohort differences can also be found when we compare biologically related individuals; that is, parents and their adult offspring measured at the same age. Figure 5 provides this comparison and once again shows that the younger generation does better on Inductive Reasoning, Spatial Orientation and Verbal Ability, but that the older generation exceeds the younger at comparable ages on Numeric ability.[5]

What are the reasons for these very substantial generational differences? Perhaps one of the most obvious reason may be found in the dramatic increase in number of years of education (see Figure 6). On average, there was an increase of 5 years of formal education from the cohort born around the turn of the century to the cohort born in 1938. Educational exposure is obviously most important to allow people to engage in those activities that are most likely to maintain mental competence. But note that the increase in average educational exposure has been leveling off. The linear increase in performance in young adulthood since earlier has therefore mostly come to a halt. Differences in educational level are also found within families with sons having more education than their father, and daughters having more education than their mother. Cohort differences might also be caused by changes in educational practice. For example, the substantial increase in Inductive Reasoning could be attributed to the discovery method used widely, while the decline in Numeric ability might be a consequence of the abandonment of number drills common in earlier times. Other reasons for these generational differences may, of course, be found in better health care, the conquest of early childhood infectious diseases, and the adoption of more healthful life styles.

DIFFERENCES IN RATE OF AGING ACROSS GENERATIONS

Finally, in this chapter, we are concerned with the question whether differences across successive generations are confined to differences in levels attained in young adulthood, or whether there are also differences in the rate of cognitive decline with advancing age. As shown in Figure 7, the answer to this question is still somewhat mixed. In this figure we show within groups age changes on two abilities from age 60 to age 81 for three successive cohorts. Note that for Inductive Reasoning there is not only increase in level at age 60, but the decline in old age has slowed down. On the other hand the data on Spatial Orientation also show increase in level across cohorts at age 60, but once the 80s are reached there is no difference; in fact the age gradient has become a bit steeper. The lesson from these data should be that generational changes are ability specific and can not be generalized for all skills and under all circumstances.

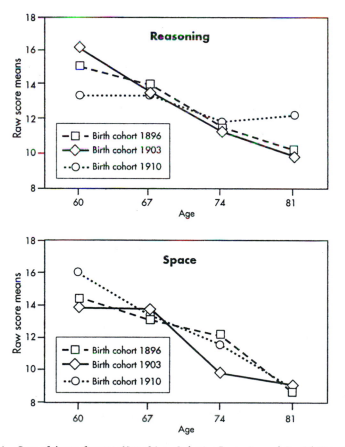

Figure 6 – Rate of change from age 60 to 81 on Inductive Reasoning and Spatial Orientation.
Adapted from Schaie, 1996.

ANTECEDENTS OF
INDIVIDUAL DIFFERENCES

Why is it that some people age faster than others? This topic is, of course, central to this volume. Here I would mention a number of variables that we have identified that are specifically relevant to the aging of behavioral competence.[3,7] First of all, it is quite clear that the absence of chronic disease is positively associated with the maintenance of intellectual abilities as we age. In addition to the obvious importance of an intact physiological infrastructure for optimal behavior, it is also clear that those free of chronic disease are at an advantage in maintaining life styles that enhance cognitive functioning.[3,8]

Secondly, maintenance of cognitive abilities into old age is enhance by living in favorable environmental circumstances, such as would be the case for persons with high socio-economic status. But in addition, involvement in activities that are complex and intellectually stimulating, such as travel, extensive reading, adult education activities, cultural activities, are all helpful in maintaining cognitive competence.

A third factor involves personality styles. Individuals who at mid-life tend to be role changes inherent in advancing age were found to be better of in maintaining high levels of competence into old age.[7,11] It seems that flexible persons are also more likely to take risks and seek high levels of intellectual stimulation.

Fourth, it helps to be married to a spouse functioning at a high level of cognitive abilities. This finding does not surprise because the spousal relationship is probably the most immediate environmental circumstance that can provide stimulating interactions.[9]

Fifth, we have implicated the maintaining of perceptual processing speed (or reaction time) as an indicator of central nervous fitness. Those individuals who remain high in perceptual speed well into old age are at an advantage because they can process information and respond in a faster manner.[10]

Finally, there is the intangible factor of how persons feel about themselves and how they perceive their own competence. Maintenance of intellectual competence into advantage age is accompanied not only by selfratings of success in life,[4] but also by perceptions of maintenance or gain in their own intellectual competence.[12]

Just as one can specify risk factors for various diseases, it is also possible to specify risk factors for the occurrence of significant cognitive decline. As part of our studies we have developed a calculus, that indicates the relative magnitude of a number of these risk factors.[4] Table 1 shows how such a calculus might proceed for five mental abilities. The first line in this table in this table indicates the average age at which one might expect to experience a significant decline on each of these abilities. Then we adjust these number by correction factors reflecting specific personal attributes. For example, for females the decline event, on average, will occur five

Table 2.2 – Parameters for predicting age at which first decline event is most likey to occur

Predictor variable	Adjustment in years				
	Verbal Meaning	Spatial Orientation	Inductive Reasoning	Number	Word Fluency
Average age of decline	67.83	62.61	64.88	64.52	63.37
Female	5.29	5.44	4.67	5.03	4.37
Education (per year above mean)	1.35	1.13	0.83	1.03	1.08
Observed decline in behavioural flexibility	-6.44	-6.20	-3.46	-5.87	-6.02
Above average success in life	2.71	4.80	2.58	1.80	2.97
Above average life satisfaction		2.30			

Positive values are added to the average estimate of age of decline, negative values are subtracted.

Adapted from Schaie (1989a).

years later than for males. The effects of education suggest that decline will occur approximately one year later for each year of education above the population mean (or conversely earlier for people with below average levels of education). Persons who have become more rigid will decline at a faster rate than those who are flexible. And, again those who have experienced above average life success will decline at a later age.

SUMMARY

In this chapter I have described the average age changes in mental abilities with age that are characteristic for normal community-dwelling persons. I have suggested that these changes are not universal in the sense that very few people decline on all mental abilities. Nevertheless, it is quite likely that by the time the 60s are reached, there will be decline on one or more abilities (typically those that have been used the least in a person's daily life). As indicated in the chapter by Willis these changes in normal persons are certainly not irreversible. However, we also know that while substantial cognitive decline prior to age 60 is usually an early indicator of a pathological process, it is only the few and fortunate who reach the late 80s without experiencing substantial decline in their intellectual competence. Within the range from the 60s to the 80s individual differences in rate of change are great and are affected by health status, genetic predisposition. and the maintenance of active and intellectually stimulation life styles.

We also suggested that there have been upward shifts in many abilities for successive cohorts over this century, and that rates of aging may have slowed for some but not all abilities. We further suggested that maintenance of high levels of intellectual of functioning can be enhanced by maintaining an intellectually challenging environment, living with an intelligent spouse, and adopting flexible personality styles. These characteristics are currently displayed primarily by the more advantaged members of our society. But interventions are available that might enhance these attributes in a broader population and markedly increase the quality of life of those persons who are willing to take a more active role in managing their own lives towards the objective of successful aging.

ACKNOWLEDGEMENT

The Seattle Longitudinal Study findings from which are reported in this chapter is currently supported by research grant R37 AG08055 from the National Institute on Aging. I am also greatly indebted for the enthusiastic support of this study by the members and staff of the Group Health Cooperative of Puget Sound.

REFERENCES

1. Schaie KW. Rigidity-flexibility and intelligence: A cross-sectional study of the adult life-span from 20 to 70. *Psychol Monogr* 1958; **72(No. 462)**:Whole No. 9

2. Schaie KW. The course of adult intellectual development. *Amer Psychol* 1994; **49**: 304-313

3. Schaie KW. Intellectual Development in Adulthood: The Seattle Longitudinal Study. New York: Cambridge University Press, 1996

4. Schaie KW. The hazards of cognitive aging. Gerontologist 1989; **29**:484-493

5. Schaie KW, Plomin R, Willis SL, Gruber-Baldini A, Dutta R. Natural cohorts: Family similarity in adult cognition. In: Sonderegger T, ed. *Psychology and aging: Nebraska Symposium on Motivation, 1991*. Lincoln, NE: University of Nebraska Press, 1992: pp 205-243

6. Willis SL. Cohort differences in cognitive aging: A sample case. In: Schaie KW, Schooler C, eds. *Social structure and aging: Psychological processes*. Hillsdale, NJ: Erlbaum, 1989: pp 94-112

7. Schaie KW. Midlife influences upon intellectual functioning in old age. *Intern J Behav Develop* 1984; **7**: 463-478

8. Gruber-Baldini AL. The impact of health and disease on cognitive ability in adulthood and old age in the Seattle Longitudinal Study [doctoral dissertation]: The Pennsylvania State University, 1991

9. Schaie KW. Psychological changes from midlife to old age: Implications for the maintenance of mental health. *Amer J Orthopsych* 1981; **51:** 199-218

10. Gruber-Baldini AL, Schaie KW, Willis SL. Similarity in married couples: A longitudinal study of mental abilities and flexibility-rigidity. *J Person Soc Psychol: Personality Processes and Individual Differences* 1995; 69:191-203

11. Schaie KW. Perceptual speed in adulthood: Cross-sectional and longitudinal studies. *Psych & Aging* 1989; 4:443-453

12. Schaie KW, Willis SL, O'Hanlon AM. Perceived intellectual performance change over seven years. *J Geront: Psychological Sciences.* 1994; **49:** P108-P118

3

LIFESTYLE RISK FACTORS FOR COGNITIVE IMPAIRMENT

Lon R. White,* Daniel J. Foley and Richard J. Havlik

* co-investigators for these analyses include H. Petrovitch, K. Masaki, G.W. Ross, D. Chiu, R. Abbott, L. Launer, P. Chyou, and J.D. Curb.

*P*oor performance on tests of cognitive function among older persons is most often attributed to 'normal aging' or to a dementing illness.[1] It is unclear to what extent the declines of normal aging are due to changes in test-taking skills following retirement, changes in family constellation, a narrowing range of daily activities outside the home, a declining interest in knowing about the world through reading and television, or a general constriction of interpersonal in teractions. Depression, delirium, stroke, and other specific diseases seem to be relatively infrequent causes of poor test performance in older persons living independently, and are distinct from dementia and normal aging as causes of poor test performance.

The findings reported here are from an ongoing epidemiologic study of dementia in aging Japanese–American men living in Honolulu.[2] Analyses will be presented addressing the relative contributions of dementia and other causes to poor cognitive test performance in this cohort. In addition, preliminary data will be presented relating to possible associations of several defined lifestyle risk factors with poor performance on tests of cognitive function, as well as with specific diagnoses of Alzheimer's disease or vascular dementia.

The Honolulu–Asia Aging Study (HAAS) is a National Institute on Aging (NIA) directed component of the Honolulu Heart Program (HHP).[3,4] The HHP is a longitudinal study of heart disease, stroke and cancer. It was established in 1965 with the enrollment, interview, and examination of 8006 Japanese–American men born in 1900 through 1919 and living on Oahu. During 1991-93 the NIA, National Heart Lung and Blood Institute (NHLBI), National Institute of Nursing Research (NINR), and the Department of Veterans Affairs (DVA) co-supported a re-examination of surviving study participants — the fourth examination of the full cohort since the project's inception. Data collection and analyses are funded through research contracts with the University of Hawaii and Kuakini Medical Center. The (4th HHP) examination included measurement of cognitive function, detection of cases of dementia by clinical evaluation, and investigation of possible factors involved in the pathogenesis of Alzheimer's disease (AD) and vascular dementia.

The HAAS was designed in cooperation with researchers from centers in Japan, Taiwan, and the United States; studies paralleling the HAAS are currently being conducted in Seattle, Hiroshima, and Taipei.[2] The major instruments used at all sites include the Cognitive Abilities Screening Instrument (CASI) and the Informant Questionnaire on Cognitive Decline in the Elderly (IQCODE), a standardized proxy interview for defining deterioration in cognitive and behavioral function.[5,6] For most analyses, poor performance on the CASI was defined as a score <75 (corresponding to a Mini-Mental State Examination score of less than 22/23); intermediate performance as between 75 and 82, and normal performance as a score of 82-100. An IQCODE score <3.25 was interpreted as indicating no apparent decline over the previous 10 years, while >3.6 was taken as strong evidence of decline, and 3.25-3.59 was considered marginal.

Of the 3734 participants tested during the 1991-93 examination cycle, 587 received a low CASI score. Eighty-one percent (n=478) of these apparently cognitively impaired received a re-evaluation 2-16 weeks later that included re-administration of the CASI to the participant and administration of the IQCODE to his 'significant other', usually his wife. Results of the relationship of IQCODE to persistently low CASI scores are shown in Table 3.1; of those for whom the IQCODE indicated a decline, 91% had a repeat CASI score that was still low. This observation supports the usefulness of informant information in predicting persistently poor CASI scores.

A sample of individuals was then selected to receive a second re-evaluation, as a result of which the individuals were classified as demented or not demented. Results were used to estimate the percent of persons meeting the stringent Diagnostic and Statistical Manual - Third Revision (DSMIIIR) criteria for dementia. The percent of persons meeting more relaxed criteria (Benson and Cummings 'clinical dementia' criteria) was also estimated for each combination. The data in Table 3.2 show

Table 3.1 — Number and percent (in brackets) distribution of IQCODE results by status of the repeated CASI: HAAS 1991-1993.

IQCODE	Number	Repeat CASI Still low	Repeat CASI Intermediate	Repeat CASI Normal
Not done	40 (100%) 190	29 (72)	6 (15)	5 (13)
No decline		88 (46)	63 (33)	39 (21)
Marginal	87	53 (61)	23 (26)	11 (13)
Decline	161	146 (91)	11 (7)	4 (2)
Total	478 (100%)	316 (66)	103 (22)	59 (12)

Table 3.1 – *Prevalence of dementia using stringent DSMIIIR diagnostic criteria and more-relaxed Cumming-Benson criteria (C-B, in brackets) according to status of the repeat CASI, by IQCODE results: HAAS 1991-1993.*

	Repeat CASI Still low	Repeat CASI Intermediate	Repeat CASI Normal
IQCOE results	DSMIIIR C-B	DSMIIIR C-B	DSMIIIR C-B
Not done	78% (78%)	0% (67%)	0% (13%)
No decline	23% (49%)	7% (22%)	0% (5%)
Marginal	60% (77%)	35% (71%)	25% (50%)
Decline	90% (95%)	80% (80%)	18% (45%)

prevalence of dementia among persons in each subgroup, defined using stringent or relaxed (in parentheses) diagnostic criteria.

We interpret these data as suggesting that a substantial proportion of persons judged to have cognitive impairment on the basis of a single screening test may not show persistently poor performance on second testing (Table 3.1). Cognitive performance at two testings, considered conjointly with the IQCODE (cognitive decline) score allows fairly efficient discrimination of dementia from cognitive impairment not attributable to a dementing illness. Most instances of persistent poor CASI performance were attributed to dementing diseases, rather than normal aging (Table 3.2).

These diagnostic maneuvers, coupled with careful sampling and statistical adjustment strategies, allowed us to generate prevalence estimates for our cohort, to adjust these estimates to the age-structure of a standard reference population (we used the 65+ population of the United States in 1990), and to compare the estimates with rates previously reported for other populations. The age-standardized prevalence of Alzheimer's disease was estimated at 4.7% (95% confidence limits (CL): 2.8-7.5). This figure was calculated with the inclusion of cases in which Alzheimer's disease was felt to be either the primary or a contributing cause. The corresponding figure for vascular dementia was 3.8% (CL: 2.1-6.4). Because many of the cases had more than a single contributing cause, the estimate of total dementia prevalence was 7.6% (CL: 5.1-10.8).

Such estimates serve two main purposes: they facilitate planning related to the development and allocation of health care resources, and they provide clues to factors that may be involved in pathogenesis. A major impetus underlying our research came from prior reports from Japan indicating higher rates of vascular dementia and lower rates of Alzheimer's disease, compared with rates in most populations of European decent. While our findings did indeed confirm a relatively high prevalence of vascular dementia among Japanese-American men living in Hawaii, rates of Alzheimer's disease approximated those previously reported from other American and European communities and were higher than estimates from most Japanese studies.[2] These observations led us to speculate that migration from Japan to Hawaii had not substantially affected the pathogenesis of vascular dementia, but was associated with an increase in the occurrence of Alzheimer's disease. The veracity of these interpretations awaits further research using cross-nationally standardized methods and end points. Ultimately, such differences or similarities in the occurrence of a specific dementing disease in genetically or environmentally varied populations could facilitate efforts to identify lifestyle factors related to cognitive decline and dementia.

We have conducted preliminary analyses of the possible associations of selected lifestyle risk factors in HAAS with: 1. very poor cognitive test scores, defined as a CASI score less than 75; 2. Alzheimer's disease; 3. vascular dementia.

Candidate risk factor information was collected during standardized interviews and examinations 20-30 years earlier. Initial analyses showed the expected strong associations of CASI test score with age and years of education. Potential associations with risk factors were examined separately for the three end points using multiple logistic or linear regression modeling. With Alzheimer's disease as the end point, the only control co-variate was age. With vascular dementia as the end point, age and history of stroke were used as the basic control co-variates. With poor CASI score as the end point (either including or excluding dementing illnesses), the regression models included age, years of education, and history of stroke. Results are summarized below:

- Alcohol consumption — no apparent associations with poor CASI score, AD, or vascular dementia;

- Coffee consumption — no apparent associations with poor CASI score, AD, or vascular dementia;

- Smoking — slight association between cigarette smoking and poor CASI score; the association became statistically non-significant after controlling for age, education, history of stroke, and systolic blood pressure;

- Years of education — not significantly associated with AD or vascular dementia; more than 5 children — marginal association with poor CASI score but not with AD or vascular dementia;

- Low-complexity occupation — association with poor CASI score but not with AD or vascular dementia;

- Traditional Japanese diet, as indicated by high intake of green tea, tofu, and miso soup — associated with Alzheimer's disease as well as with poor CASI score not attributed to either AD or vascular dementia; not associated with vascular dementia;

- Lower body mass index — marginally associated with AD;

- Higher density of persons/bedroom in home — marginally associated with poor CASI score but not with AD or vascular dementia;
- No statistically significant associations were noted for marital status, number of marriages, number of siblings, birth order, religion, black tea consumption, total dietary calories, total dietary protein, total dietary fat, percent dietary protein from animal sources, frequency of ingesting ham/bacon or cheese/margarine or milk or seaweed, or years worked on a sugarcane or pineapple plantation.

Two constitutional factors — not listed above, but that might indirectly reflect lifestyle factors — have received in-depth examination as influencers of cognitive function. These are a measure of pulmonary function (rate of forced expiratory volume (in liters) in one second (FEV1)) and blood pressure.[7,8]

Lifestyle and environmental factors are well-known contributors to the quality of lung function over the lifespan. Behaviors, such as smoking and exercise, can affect pulmonary function considerably as can air-quality in the neighborhood, home and workplace. A recently published analysis of the relationship between FEV1 performance measured at base line and CASI performance measured 25 years later showed a significant positive association.[7] Basically, those under the median of 2.8 liters per second for FEV1 had a mean CASI score of 79.8 versus a mean CASI score of 85.4 among those above the median ($p < 0.0001$ for trend). However, when the analyses were adjusted for possible confounding by way of differences in age, education, prevalence of stroke, manual versus non-manual occupational history, hours spent in sedentary activities per day, height, generation, and ability to speak Japanese, the relationship was substantially weakened but remained significant with CASI scores of 82.9 versus 84.1 for the lower and upper half of FEV1 values, respectively ($p < 0.03$ for trend). This relationship between FEV1 and CASI score was stronger among those under 55 years of age at base line. This may suggest an interaction related to FEV1 scores' association with age and mortality or both.[9] In essence, for each deciliter increase in FEV1 there was a corresponding increase of about one eighth of a point change in the CASI score, all else being equal ($p < 0.05$). In the absence of a base line test of cognitive function, however, there is uncertainty as to whether poorer pulmonary function over the lifespan corresponds with poorer cognitive function over the same period. On the other hand, the findings may represent 'the interesting possibility that accelerated aging of the lung might predict accelerated aging of the brain'.[7]

The effect of elevated blood pressure (BP) on subsequent stroke is well known, and treatment of systolic hypertension as a preventive approach has been established.[10] Although most individuals require medications for effective BP lowering, in some cases attainment of BP in the normal range is possible through a regimen of weight loss, decreased salt intake and exercise.[11] In addition to stroke there have been reports of elevated BP being associated with characteristic changes on brain Magnetic Resonance Imaging (MRI), called white matter hyperintensities, which probably represent the effect of silent small blood vessel disease in the brain.[12] Although these cerebral findings have not been established as a definitive link with poorer performance on cognitive function testing, there has been a report from Hawaii suggesting a relationship of neuropathologically determined small vessel disease with elevated BP.[13]

In the well-known Framingham community study of cardiovascular risk factors, which has a similar longitudinal design to the HAAS, it has been demonstrated that BPs measured about 20 years prior to cognitive function testing have been associated with more recent poorer function.[14] However, the relationship attenuated dramatically as the measurement of BP occurred closer to the time of cognitive testing. Because of the importance of this observation both for understanding pathophysiology as well as potential effects in preventing cognitive decline for the individual and the larger population, it was decided to replicate this observation within the HAAS. The confirmatory results have been published,[8] but the methods and findings are instructive and will be summarized here.

The goal of the analysis was to determine the possible effect of mid-life BP on later life cognitive function. As indicated earlier in the chapter, a number of cardiovascular risk factors had been measured at periodic examinations in approximately 1965, 1968 and 1971 as well as at the time of cognitive function testing in 1991-93. Specifically, BP level was determined as the average of three systolic BP measurements at each of the examinations. These values were grouped into BP categories of low (≤110 mmHg.), normal (110-139), borderline (140-159), and high (3160). An individual had to fall into one of the categories during at least two examinationss to be assigned to a category. If those BP conditions did not occur, the individual was classified as 'mixed' BP. A history of use of antihypertensive medication was determined, but the classification of subjects was done by the absolute BP level. The previously described CASI score was divided into three categories, because the distribution of the CASI scores was not Gaussian. A good score was 92-100, intermediate 82-<92, and poor <82. The poor cutoff identified approximately 30% of the population as lowest scorers. This is a less affected subpopulation than previously identified by the score below 75, which represented only about 16% of the population. Besides education and age, which have been shown to be major predictors of cognitive function, there was substantial information available about cardiovascular risk factors and diagnoses such as stroke, defined by ongoing hospital surveillance and a diagnostic consensus process in this study. Multiple logistic regression was used to evaluate the relationship between the categories of systolic BP blood pressure and cognitive impairment with control for confounders.

With higher categories of systolic BP the risk of intermediate and poor compared to good cognitive function increased accordingly and in a significant manner (Table 3.3). For every 10 mmHg increment of systolic BP the risk of poor cognitive function increased 9%. This was true even after adjustment for prevalent stroke, coronary heart disease and an indicator of peripheral vascular disease, although the

Table 3.3 – *Relationship (odds ratio [95% confidence interval] of mid-life systolic blood pressure to late-life cognitive function in men participating in the Honolulu Asia Aging Study (1991-1993), Follow-up of the Honolulu Heart Program (1965-1971).*

Midlife blood pressure*	No. of respondents	Cognitive Function[†]			
		Model 1[‡]		Model 2[§]	
		Intermediate	Poor	Intermediate	Poor
Low	368	1.0	1.0	1.0	1.0
Normal	2240	1.32 (1.03-1.71)	1.29 (0.94-1.76)	1.31 (1.00-1.72)	1.23 (0.88-1.71)
Borderline	646	1.23 (0.90-1.68)	1.33 (0.92-1.94)	1.22 (0.89-1.66)	1.21 (0.82-1.79)
Mixed	251	1.69 (1.10-2.61)	1.72 (1.03-2.86)	1.60 (1.02-2.50)	1.48 (0.89-2.46)
High	229	1.81 (1.11-2.95)	2.45 (1.42-4.25)	1.73 (1.04-2.87)	2.11 (1.22-3.66)
Trend		P<0.03	P<0.001	P<0.05	P<0.02

* Low indicates <110 mmHg; normal 110-139 mmHg; borderline 140-159 mmHg; and high ≥160mm Hg. A positive history was assigned if a subject had a blood pressure that fell within these limits in two of the first three examinations (1965-1971); mixed indicates no pattern or missing data on two visits.

1 Measured by the 100-point Cognitive Abilities Screening Instrument (CASI). A CASI score 392 indicates good performance; <92-82 intermediate performance; and <82 poor performance.

2 Controlling for education and age.

§ Controlling for education, age and prevalent stroke; quartiles of the ankle-brachial index; and coronary heart disease in 1992; n=3590.

Adapted from Launer et al. JAMA 1995

relationship was diminished somewhat by this analysis (Model 2 - Table 3.3). Such an analytic result provides indirect evidence that associated cardiovascular disease might play a mediating role in some but not all of the observed BP-cognitive function relationships. When cases of dementia (both Alzheimer's disease and vascular dementia), as defined above, were excluded from the analysis, the BP-cognitive function association persisted. This observation suggests that the relationship might indeed be important for the cognitive impairment that is seen with usual aging and not simply indicative of a demented subgroup. The practical inference is that there is a need for middle-life BP screening and treatment as a potential lifestyle preventive measure for cognitive impairment in old age.

There are aspects of other analytic results that require some qualification. First, diastolic BP measured during the same earlier time period did not predict later poor cognitive function. It is known that diastolic BP is a good predictor of coronary heart disease at younger ages. However, the stiffening of blood vessels through probable loss of elasticity and hardening of the ground substance in the vessel wall, which frequently accompanies usual aging, results in a lower diastolic BP at older ages. Because of these age-related changes, any potential relationship may become distorted by this other process. Of course, there are other good reasons to measure and treat elevated diastolic BP. However, more importantly for the geriatrician evaluating older patients, neither current systolic nor diastolic BP was related to concurrently assessed cognitive function. In fact it appeared that a relatively low systolic BP (<110) was associated with the highest risk of poor cognitive function. There seemed to be a threshold below which the level was associated with poorer cognitive functioning.

There are several possible explanations for the well-known phenomenon of risk factors that had been potent predictors of disease when measured in earlier life becoming less robust when assessed in later life. One possibility is that the level of the risk factor (such as BP) may be modulated by other diseases and other age-related frailties, leading to a distortion of its true relationships with the condition of interest. Another explanation is that with advancing age, disease end points become more common and less discreetly associated with a single pathogenic mechanism, making the risk factor-disease relationship less apparent. Two other intuitively appealing possibilities are:

1. The identification of a risk factor in earlier life may be a better indicator of the duration and consistency of exposure than identification of the same factor in late life.

2. Those persons still alive into their later years despite long exposure to an important risk factor may be selected for resistance to that factor, or may have survived because the level of exposure has not been constant or has diminished.

The situation is further complicated by the fact that older individuals are likely to have accumulated so much atherosclerosis and arteriosclerosis that stresses or additional risk factor exposures that would have had no effect in earlier life may precipitate a serious or fatal event. This idea suggests that even though the relationship between stroke or infarction and a risk factor measured in late life may be less clear, the consequences of an increase in exposure to the factor may be more devastating than had been the case at an earlier age. It is quite appropriate, as indicated by the successful Systolic Hypertension in the Elderly Program, that older persons with elevated systolic BP should be treated to lower BP at a minimum to prevent stroke.[10] Indeed, it might be important in preventing cognitive decline; however, therapeutic efficacy for cognition has not been proven with a controlled clinical trial. What is more evident from this research is the need for lifelong preventive measures to assure optimal cognitive function at older ages.

Overall, these findings from the HAAS suggest a complex pattern of relationships between base line variables and outcomes. Because the study is being done in a homogeneous ethnic group with a probable different mix of vascular and non-vascular factors from other US populations, the results might not be broadly generalizable. However, they do implicate mid-life systolic BP and forced expiratory volume, possibly related to smoking, as potential risk factors for cognitive impairment. However, these preliminary analyses in the HAAS fail to implicate alcohol, coffee drinking and several other factors as having an independent influence on low cognitive function or dementia in late life. The only lifestyle factors showing a significant association with a specific dementing illness were high dietary intake of green tea, tofu, and miso soup – all characteristic of a traditional Japanese diet. One interesting possibility is that phytoestrogens contained in the tofu might be affecting neuronal plasticity in an adverse way. This might occur through competition for estrogen receptors on neurons. Estrogen is thought by many to have beneficial effects on neuronal plasticity and brain function.[15] The biologic significance and epidemiologic validity of these associations is under investigation. The challenge will be to utilize research in this population and others to identify potential strategies for preventing cognitive decline in later life.

REFERENCES

1. Colsher PL, Wallace RB. Epidemiologic considerations in studies of cognitive function in the elderly: methodology and nondementing acquired dysfunction. *Epidemiol Rev* 1991; **13:** 1-27.

2. White LR. Toward a program of cross-cultural research on the epidemiology of Alzheimer's disease. *Curr Sci* 1992; **63:** 456-469.

3. Kagan A, Harris BR, Winkelstein W *et al.* Epidemiologic studies of coronary heart disease and stroke in Japanese men living in Japan, Hawaii and California: demographic, physical, dietary, and biochemical characteristics. *J Chron Dis* 1974; **27:** 345-364.

4. White LR, Petrovitch H, Ross GW *et al.* Prevalence of dementia in older Japanese-American men in Hawaii: The Honolulu-Asia Aging Study. *JAMA* In press. (???Author if now pub, pls give details)

5. Teng EL, Hasegawa K, Homma A *et al.* The Cognitive Abilities Screening Instrument (CASI): a practical test for cross-cultural epidemiological studies of dementia. *Int Psychogeriatr* 1994; **6:** 45-58.

6. Jorm AF, Scott R, Cullen JS *et al.* Performance on the Informant Questionnaire on Cognitive Decline in the Elderly (IQCODE) as a screening test for dementia. *Psych Med* 1991; **21:** 785-790.

7. Chyou P, White LR, Yano K. *et al.* Pulmonary function measures as predictors and correlates of cognitive functioning in later life. *Am J Epidemiol* 1996; **143:** 750-6.

8. Launer LJ, Masaki K, Petrovitch H *et al.* The association between midlife blood pressure levels and late-life cognitive function: The Honolulu-Asia Aging Study. *JAMA* 1995; **274:**1846-1851.

9. Rodriguez BL, Masaki K, Burchfiel C *et al.* Pulmonary function decline and 17-year total mortality: the Honolulu Heart Program. *Am J Epidemiol* 1994;**140:** 398-408.

10. SHEP Cooperative Research Group. Prevention of stroke by antihypertensive drug treatment in older persons with isolated systolic hypertension. Final results of the Systolic Hypertension in the Elderly Program (SHEP). *JAMA* 1994; **265:** 3255-3264.

11. Applegate WB, Miller ST, Elam JT *et al.* Nonpharmacologic intervention to reduce blood pressure in older patients with mild hypertension. *Arch Intern Med* 1992; **152:**1162-1166.

12. van Swieten JC, Geyskes GG, Derix MMA *et al.* Hypertension in the elderly is associated with white matter lesions and cognitive decline. *Ann Neurol* 1991; **30:** 825-830.

13. Reed D, Jacobs Jr DR, Hayashi T *et al.* A comparison of lesions in small intracerebral arteries among Japanese men in Hawaii and Japan. *Stroke* 1994; **25:** 60-65.

14. Elias MF, Wolf PA, D'Agostino RB *et al.* Untreated blood pressure level is inversely related to cognitive functioning: the Framingham Study. *Am J Epidemiol.* 1993; **138:** 353-364.

15. Fillit H. Future therapeutic developments of estrogen use. *J Clin Pharmacol* 1995; **35:** 255-285.

4

EDUCATION AND DEPRESSION AS RISK FACTORS FOR COGNITIVE DECLINE

Robert Katzman

DEPRESSION AND DEMENTIA

One of the extraordinary advances during the past 20 years or so is the marked improvement in our ability to diagnose dementia. Clinical series carried out in the 1970s indicated that when patients were examined again after 4 or 5 years as many as a third of the patients had been misdiagnosed as having been demented, whereas recent reports show that less than 5% are misdiagnosed today.

A study in the 1970s from the Maudsley, a major psychiatric referral hospital in London, UK, showed that patients who had been diagnosed with Alzheimer's disease of the presenile type, the classic form with onset before the age of 65, were correctly diagnosed in only 70% of cases.[1] The other 30%, when re-examined at least 4 years later, were found to have other disorders, notably depression misdiagnosed as dementia.

In the 1970s a number of psychiatrists started to look at the question of what was called pseudodementia, i.e. patients who were depressed and showed memory changes and usually with a mild degree of cognitive deficit which could be reversed on treatment of the depression. Most of these patients had a prior history of severe depression and Folstein & McHugh[2] thought this should be termed a dementia in depression.

In 1980 the American Psychiatric Association published the third edition of their diagnostic and statistical manual (DSMIII) that listed criteria for diagnosing various conditions. It was a very important event in this field because prior to the DSMIII there were only general descriptions but not operational ones. The DSMIII criteria played a major role in that we can now diagnose these two conditions, dementia and depression, without much problem in distinguishing them. The criteria for diagnosing dementia are a loss of intellectual abilities which interfere with something one does, the social or occupational functioning of an individual; impairment of memory; and impairment of at least one other area of cognition in one who is alert and awake. Major depression depends not only upon the depressed mood but on the presence of additional symptoms, such as change in weight, change in sleep pattern, fatigue and suicidal thoughts. When these criteria are followed, the problem of differentiating dementia from depression disappears.

It turns out that if you look at people who have only depressed mood, i.e. just dysphoria, that dysphoria is much more common than major depression. This was pointed out by Blazer in a study in a population near Durham, North Carolina in 1980.[3] In a more recent study from the same area but a different population, Blazer et al[4] pointed out that in the elderly (but not in younger individuals with depression) there is a higher occurrence of depressive symptomatology in those who have cognitive impairment, using a standardized test for depressive symptoms: 17% of those with cognitive impairment showed depression compared with 8% of those without cognitive impairment.

Chapter 3 refers to a series of studies from Europe called European re-analysis, although 7 of the 11 studies were from the US5. Data from case-controlled studies of Alzheimer's patients versus normal controls were combined. Because these investigators were able to put together 11 of these studies, many of which had about 100 Alzheimer's patients and a 100 nondemented subjects, over 1000 subjects were obtained in each category. With the statistical power this provided they could look at odds ratios and the risk factors in these well-diagnosed Alzheimer's patients. As mentioned in Chapter 3, smoking emerged as a protective factor but was not statistically significant. A family history of dementia was the most important predictor for dementia. Surprisingly, depression occurring after the age of 70 was reported in a series to be a risk factor for Alzheimer's disease, which presents the question, 'is this a risk factor or is it the first symptom?' The lack of an answer is a persistent problem when considering risk factors in Alzheimer's disease.

Alzheimer's is a chronic disease. There are initiation factors that may occur in some people at birth, that is initial genetic susceptibility in almost half the cases. There are unknown promoting factors, with the exception of age and head trauma. Then there is clearly, as we know from autopsy studies, a preclinical phase in which there are changes in the brain but no symptoms. Then clinical symptoms appear and although we now have good critera that allow an accurate diagnosis, this can only be made months to years after the first symptoms. We do not really know what the first clinical symptoms are and it may be that depression or a change of lifestyle at this point may be misinterpreted as a risk factor for dementia.

EDUCATION AS A RISK FACTOR

In 1988 Mortimer[6] argued that the clinical diagnosis of dementia of the Alzheimer's type results from a combination of physiological and psychosocial processes, and that the psychosocial factors act primarily to reduce the margin of intellectual reserve to a level where more modest level of brain pathology results in a diagnosable dementia. Two testable hypotheses were proposed, that the psychosocial risk factors will have their strongest association in late onset Alzheimer's disease of mild to moderate severity, and that low pre-morbid intelligence hastens the clinical diagnosis of dementia of the Alzheimer type.

George Beadle, a Nobel laureate, who started the revolution in biochemical genetics in the 1940s and later became president of the University of Chicago, died of Alzheimer's disease at the age of 86. Dr Beadle was clearly a highly educated and intelligent individual. Every individual is susceptible to developing Alzheimer's disease, but a discussion of risk factors should focus on populations.

PREVALENCE STUDIES

I have been involved in a study of dementia in the Jin An district of Shanghai with the Shanghai Institute of Mental Health led by Dr Mingyuan Zhang, and expertise in neurology, neuropsychology and psychiatry provided by the University of California, San Diego.[7] The goal was to provide training in the diagnosis of dementia along Western lines. The population sample was stratified and the very old were over-sampled. The original objective was to enrol 1500 people in each of 3 age groups – 55-64, 65-74 and 75+ – and while this was not quite achieved, the figures came close, with a total of 5055 individuals. Few of the individuals have been to school, a factor that had not been appreciated at the start of the study. Some 27% had had no formal education whatsoever. In modern China this is not a direct reflection of one's occupation or lifestyle because, during the cultural revolution which lasted about 10 years, society was reversed and those with the highest level of education were sent out into the countryside to work in the fields.

During the 1950s the Chinese government attempted to provide adult literacy education, but our Shanghai sample would suggest this did not work. On the Chinese version of the Mini Mental Status Exam (CMMS), only 9% of the sample could read a simple phrase.[8] Also, surprisingly, most could not copy an intersecting pentagon, one of the tasks in the exam and apparently if you do not learn to copy as a child, you will not complete the task when presented with it at 75 years old!

As would be predicted, the level of education had a marked effect on the mental status test scores. We divided the cohort into 3 groups: one with no education; one with 1-6 years of education; and the third with more than 6 years at school and including a couple with PhDs or MDs. Most of those in the third group as well as the 5-64 year olds achieved a good score on the CMMS; those aged 75 years and over and who had received some education, a somewhat lower score. However, in general these individuals performed similarly to a Western population.

Those who had received no education had very different scores and even the 55 year olds scored only 21-22. Therefore, for clinical evalution, we decided to select individuals from the highest education group who scored below 24 and in the group with no education, those with scores below 21. We also took a 5% random sample of the entire population.

To diagnose dementia we applied a number of tests similar to those used in the US.[9] We used some psychometric tests in addition to mental status tests, including the number of animals that could be named in a period of time. For memory tests we used physical objects as a way of avoiding cultural bias in deciding what words to use in the memory tests (the Fuld Object Memory Test). The digit span subtest of the WAIS worked quite well as it would appear that in a modern society, even if you cannot read or draw, you need to learn to count. It was difficult to find an appropriate test of constructional and visual-spatial awareness and we had to use the children's version of the block design, a subtest of WISC, to test this cognitive function. Measures of functional change were also applied.

In the two younger age groups, 55-64 and 64-74 years old, there were few individuals with dementia and no clear relationship to education. However, in the 75-84 year old group, as predicted by Mortimer,[6] there was a marked education effect. Among the women, the prevalence of dementia in those with no education was 18%, in those with elementary education 12%, and in those with middle grade education 4%. Even at the age of 85 years, education has an effect, although this is not great. As we were concerned that the relationship identified may have been an artifact of our misdiagnosing dementia in patients who tested poorly because they had not attended school, we did a factor analysis to determine what predicted the diagnosis of dementia. The CMMS did but it was markedly affected by education; however, history questions and a functional status questionnaire, the Pfeffer functional scale,[10] also predicted the diagnosis of dementia quite well and these were free of an education effect.

In our clinical evelution, history was obtained from an informant. Two instrumental activities of daily living scales were used, and one, designed in Leisure World in Irvine, California, by Robert Pfeffer, was quite powerful. We created a Chinese version of the questionnaire, for example substituting a question asking if you could handle a cheque book, for one asking about coupons. If we used just the history questions and the Pfeffer scale as a measure of dementia, we saw the same education effect.[11]

In a similar study in Bordeaux, France, including a number of illiterates, the same education effect was found.[12] With a logistic regression to adjust for age and gender, the relative risk of developing dementia in those without education was two-fold, about the same ratio as obtained in Shanghai. In most Western samples there will not be a large group who are illiterate, but when comparing primary versus secondary education, a trend is still seen.

INCIDENCE STUDIES

In incidence studies the concern that poor performance by illiterates might be mistaken for dementia is eliminated since changes in scores in individuals during follow-up are determined in order to identify new cases of dementia. In one incidence study,[13] a section of North Manhattan that was one-third white, one-third black and one-third Hispanic was studied, and 593 non-demented subjects were followed. It was found that less than 8 years of education doubled the risk of developing dementia and that a low, unskilled occupation doubled the risk. If an individual had low education and a low occupation, the risk of developing dementia was tripled.

Numerous other studies have reported similar effects of low education and low occupation, a notable exception being the Framingham cohort.[14]

We interpret these findings from many groups and locales as indicating that if you have been educated and then employed in a cognitively demanding occupation, the onset of dementia is delayed for 5-7 years. If the prevalence of dementia is plotted against age using the log scale for prevalence, a direct relationship is seen,[15] with the prevalence doubling every 5 years of age. Thus, if the onset of dementia can be delayed 5 years, the number of cases will be halved.

We have also carried out an incidence study in Shanghai and in preliminary analysis of the 75-84 year old age group, a much higher incidence of dementia was found in illiterates than in those who had received education. We also found a fall off in the incidence of dementia in the very oldest group with no education. It is as if those who were predisposed to dementia because of, for example, their genetic susceptibility and who were not educated had all developed dementia and the incidence was declining, whereas in the other education groups the incidence continues to increase. This finding supports the Mortimer hypothesis but unfortunately the number of subjects in the very advanced age group is too small to give it any real weight.

CONCLUSION

The data from the Shanghai and Bordeaux studies support the Mortimer hypothesis, that early education increases brain reserve, thereby delaying by about 5 years the onset of cognitive impairment in those developing dementing disorders. It remains to be determined if education is a surrogate for other childhood deprivations or whether the effect of education is modified by later cognitive activity.

REFERENCES

1. Ron MA, Toone BK, Garralda ME, Lishman WA. Diagnostic accuracy in presenile dementia. *Br J Psychiat* 1979; **134**: 161-168.

2. Folstein MF, McHugh PR, Katzman R, Terry RD, Bick KL. Dementia syndrome of depression. *Alzheimer's Dis* 1978; **7**: 87-93.

3. Blazer D, Williams CD. Epidemiology of dysphoria and depression in an elderly population. *Am J Psychiat* 1980; **137(4)**: 439-444.

4. Blazer D, Burchett B, Service C, George LK. The association of age and depression among the elderly: an epidemiologic exploration. *J Gerontol* 1991; **46(6):** M210-215.

5. Van Duijn CM, Stijnen T, Hofman A. Risk factors for Alzheimer's disease: Overview of the EURODEM Collaborative Re-Analysis of Case-Control Studies. *Int J Epidemiol* 1991; **20(supp2):** S4-12.

6. Mortimer JA. Do psychological risk factors contribute to Alzheimer's disease? In: Henderson AS, Henderson JS (eds) *Etiology of Dementia of Alzheimer's Type,* (Author??? Publisher???), 1988, pp 39-52.

7. Yu ES, Liu WT, Levy MY *et al.* Cognitive impairment among elderly adults in Shanghai, China. *J Gerontol* 1989; 44: S97-106.

8. Katzman R, Zhang MY, Ouang YQ *et al.* A Chinese version of the Mini-Mental State Examination: impact of illiteracy in a Shanghai dementia survey. *J Clin Epidemiol* 1988; **41:** 971-978.

9. Zhang M, Katzman R, Jin H *et al.* The prevalence of dementia and Alzheimer's disease (AD) in Shanghai, China: Impact of age, gender and education. *Ann Neurol* 1990; 27: 428-437.

10. Pfeffer RI, Kurosaki TT, Harrah CH et al. Measurement of functional activities in older adults in the community. *J Gerontol* 1982; 37: 323-329.

11. Hill Lr, Klauber M, Katzman R *et al.* Functional status, education and the diagnosis of dementia in the Shanghai survey. *Neurology* 1993; 43; 138-145.

12. Dartigues JF, Gagnon M, Michel P et al. Le programme de recherche Paquid sur l'epidemiologie de la demence methodes et resultats initiaux. *Rev Neurol (Paris)* 1991: **147(3):** 225-230.

13. Stern Y, Gurland B, Tatemichi TK, Tang MX, Wilder D, Mayeux R. Influence of education and occupation on the incidence of Alzheimer's disease. *JAMA* 1994; 271: 1004-1010.

14. Katzman R. Views and reviews: Education and the prevalence of dementia and Alzheimer's disease. *Neurology* 1993; **43:** 13-20.

15. Jorm AF, Korten AE, Henderson SA. The prevalence of dementia: A quantitative integration of the literature. *Acta Psychiat Scand* 1987; **76:** 464-479.

5

PHYSICAL ACTIVITY AND COGNITIVE FUNCTION IN OLD AGE

Eleanor M. Simonsick

Maintaining independence well into old age is a highly desired and valued objective at the individual and societal levels. Preserving cognitive function - memory, reasoning, and information processing skills - is essential for the maintenance of independent living. This chapter reviews the potential of physical activity as a strategy for preventing cognitive decline.

In Figure 5.1, Harry calls to his wife, "Mildred, I'm going for a jog, I'm feeling a little stupid today". At present, there is insufficient empirical data on the relationship between physical activity and cognition to determine whether Harry has the right idea; it remains unknown if going out for a run or doing any physical activity on a habitual basis will improve intellectual functioning. This chapter begins with a review of the current state of the literature relevant to the relationship between physical activity and cognitive function in old age. The review addresses the following questions:

1. Are physical activity and cognitive function associated?

2. What is the nature of this association?; Is it direct, indirect, causative, spurious?

3. What are the underlying mechanisms of the association?; What are the biologic and physiologic connections?

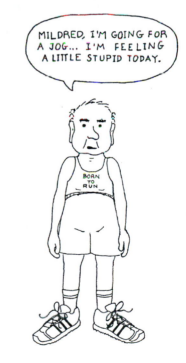

Figure 5.1

4. Can physical activity improve cognitive function? (Although the objective is preventing or minimizing decline in old age, in actual practice, research experiments have been designed with improvement as the outcome.) If activity can improve cognition, for whom is it most effective and in what areas or dimensions does it operate?

Next, empirical findings from an epidemiologic study of the cross-sectional and longitudinal relationships between physical activity and cognitive function are presented. The chapter concludes with recommendations for future research.

ARE PHYSICAL ACTIVITY AND COGNITIVE FUNCTION ASSOCIATED?

At the population level, in both large and small scale studies using national, community, volunteer, and convenience samples, physical activity and fitness are positively and inactivity, negatively associated with cognitive function. At any one point in time, persons with higher levels of physical activity or fitness perform better, on average, on tests of intellectual function than persons who are less active or less fit.[1-4] These relationships have been observed in studies examining high level cognitive functioning and in those examining the absence of dementia or poor functioning.

This type of evidence, however, is insufficient to demonstrate the value of physical activity as a preventive strategy. First, on the basis of cross-sectional data, it is equally likely that good cognition promotes physical activity as physical activity promotes good cognition. Second, several associations identified in population studies indicate that the relationship between physical activity and cognitive function may be complex and could be largely indirect. For example, cognitive performance is strongly and consistently positively related to educational attainment.[5-7] Education and physical activity are also positively correlated – the proportion physically active is typically higher in older persons with high levels of education than in those with less education; average years of school and the proportion graduating from high school is higher among the physically active than the non-active.[8-11] Thus cognitive function and physical activity may be related only as a function of education.

Similarly, poor health is negatively associated with cognitive function. Older persons in poor health tend to perform less well on cognitive tests than those who are not sick.[12,13] Persons in poor health tend not to be very physically active or physically fit either. Consequently, the relationship between cognitive function and physical activity could be a function of health status.

Depressive symptoms are also negatively associated with cognitive function, at the population and individual levels.[9,14] Depression has a negative impact on test performance.[15,16] Inactivity and depressive symptoms are also strongly correlated with persons exhibiting high levels of depressive symptoms having low activity levels.[17-19] Thus personal effect, as well, may help explain the association between measured cognition and activity.

While the associations described above suggest that physical activity and cognitive function may be only spuriously related, there exist several plausible biologic and physiologic connections between physical activity and cognitive function that support the potential for a causative association.

Underlying mechanisms

The possible mechanisms underlying the association between physical activity and cognitive function can be classified as indirect and direct. The indirect mechanisms are largely disease related (Fig. 5.2).

Physical activity has been found in population studies to be associated with lower blood pressure and lower rates of hypertension.[20] In intervention studies and exercise trials, blood pressure has been found to decrease following a program of physical activity.[21] Hypertension is a major risk factor for stroke[22] and stroke can have devastatingly negative effects on cognitive function. To the degree that physical activity can prevent stroke, physical activity can prevent stroke-related cognitive decline.

Physical activity is among the most effective strategies for the reduction of obesity and maintanence of a healthy body weight.[23] Obesity, particularly in the abdominal region, is a major risk factor for adult-onset diabetes,[24,25] which in turn is a risk factor for vascular disease. Vascular disease is a major contributor to cognitive decline.[26] By preventing, delaying the onset, and/or reducing the severity of vascular disease (either through the reduction of obesity or other vascular disease risk factors), physical activity can theorectically prevent vascular-related cognitive decline.

Indirect Mechanisms

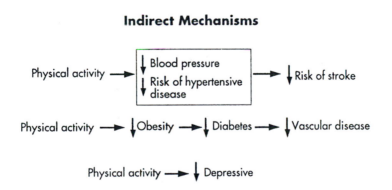

Figure 5.2

Basic Experimental Design

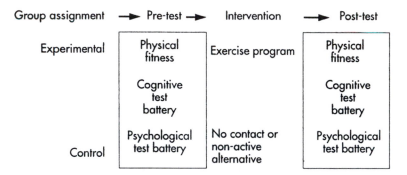

Figure 5.3

Physical activity has been found in some studies to reduce depressive symptoms in severe to moderately depressed older adults.[27] Thus physical activity may be effective in reducing cognitive deficits related to depressed affect and other mood disturbances.

In summary, physical activity has tremendous potential to prevent decline in cognitive function in old age, indirectly through its effect on risk factors for several diseases and conditions that deleteriously affect cognitive function. The evidence for an indirect effect alone is strong enough to recommend exercise as a primary preventive strategy. Whether physical activity influences cognitive function independent of disease processes remains an important question particularly for persons in good health and at low risk of developing hypertension, vascular disease, stroke, and other chronic conditions.

Two direct mechanisms through which physical activity may influence cognitive function have been proposed - improved oxidative capacity of the brain and direct stimulation of the central nervous system.[3,28,29] Fitness promoting physical activity improves the oxidative capacity of multiple systems including the cerebral region. In healthy older persons, does this improved capacity translate into improved cognitive function? Similarly, does exercise–related stimulation of the central nervous system have an impact on cognitive processes?

The major approach to addressing these issues has been through controlled experiments. Figure 5.3 shows the basic elements of experimental design. Volunteers, typically healthy, are assigned, ideally at random, to two or more groups, at least one experimental and one control. To assess baseline status, all participants, independent of group assignment, are administered a cognitive test battery and usually additional questions to determine group comparability. The experimental group(s) then receives some type of physical activity intervention. The intervention may be home- or center-based or a combination. The type and intensity of the activity, the frequency and duration of exercise sessions, as well as the length of the intervention trial can vary substantially from study to study. The control group(s) either has no contact with investigators until the end of the experimental trial or receives a non-active intervention. At the end of the intervention period, the cognitive battery is re-administered and test scores are compared.

Results from controlled experiments have been inconsistent and somewhat equivocal with regard to the value of exercise training for improving cognitive function.[28,30-37] Inconsistent findings stem largely from variations in design across studies (e.g. variations in the exercise intervention, nature of the subject population, dimension of cognition assessed) and a variety of methodologic problems. The most common limitations include:

1. Study samples too small to detect significant improvement;

2. Study samples with a large proportion of persons with limited potential for improvement or who have not experienced substantial decline, such as those younger than age 60 years, the exceptionally fit, intelligent and well educated;

3. Inappropriate test batteries – inclusion of cognitive tests that tap dimensions of crystallized intelligence such as word fluency, which remain fairly stable with increasing age.

Studies in which a positive effect for activity has been found, that is where the exercise intervention group shows statistically significant improvement relative to the control group(s), have generally contained the following elements:

1. A fitness improving exercise regimen;

2. Subjects aged 65 years and older who are poorly educated;

3. Cognitive function tests that involve processing speed as a major component.

In summary, for persons at risk, physical activity and exercise appear to be effective for primary and secondary prevention of cognitive decline associated with a wide variety of health conditions. In relatively healthy older persons, physical activity may contribute to the maintenance of and possible improvement in the processing speed component of cognitive function, particularly for the very old and poorly educated. Obviously, much more work in this area remains in order to more fully understand what physical activity can do.

PRELIMINARY FINDINGS FROM THE NEW HAVEN EPESE

Preliminary findings from an epidemiologic study are presented to illustrate some of the relationships between physical activity and cognitive function described above and the methodologic difficulties inherent in this type of research. The data come

Table 5.1 – Crude association between physical activity and cognitive function : New Haven EPESE

Level of physical activity	Number	Mean MMSE[1] score	Percent with good score[2]
Follow-up 3			
High	288	25.6***	76.0***
Moderate	549	26.2***	78.9***
Low	795	24.4	65.9
Follow-up 6			
High	281	26.3***	80.4***
Moderate	382	26.0***	79.1**
Low	684	24.9	70.0

[1] Mini-Mental State Examination
[2] Score 24 to 30 on MMSE
**p<0.01; ***p<0.001; p=probability of a difference between high or moderate activity versus low.

from the New Haven site of the Established Populations for Epidemiologic Studies of the Elderly (EPESE).[38] This study was initiated in 1982 with annual follow-up contact for 6 years through 1988. At the third annual follow-up the Mini-Mental State Examination (MMSE), a well-validated test of cognitive function primarily used as a screen for dementia, was administered.[39,40] Physical activity level was also assessed at that time. Three years later, at the sixth follow-up, the MMSE and the physical activity questions were re-administered.

The original study population consisted of a random sample of 2812 men and women aged 65 years and older stratified by housing type (public and private housing for the elderly and general community housing). Men and persons residing in either public or private elderly housing were oversampled. The majority of analyses that followed the study population consisted of only those persons in the original sample who were still living and were interviewed at follow-up six, who had valid MMSE scores and known physical activity status at both follow-ups three and six, and who had known education and health status and a valid score on the Center for Epidemiologic Studies-Depression (CES-D)[41] scale at follow-up six. Nine hundred and ninety-three persons died and 148 persons refused or were unavailable for the sixth follow-up interview. Of the remaining 1671 potential respondents, 173 had proxy interviews and an additional 272 had incomplete data on the variables of interest. Thus the final study population consisted of 1226 persons aged 71 years and older at the sixth follow-up with complete data on all measures examined.

Table 5.1 presents the crude association between physical activity level and cognitive function at the third and sixth follow-ups. Physical activity was classified into three levels – high, moderate, and low. 'High' consists of persons who, at a minimum, reported playing sports or doing physical exercise 'often', moderate consists of persons who walked 'often', and 'low' consists of persons who did very little.

Cognitive function was examined in two ways – mean MMSE scores and percent with a good score were computed for each of the activity groups. Scores on the MMSE can range from 0 to 30 with lower scores indicating poorer function. Scores of 24 or above were considered 'good'.

At both follow-ups three and six, the high and moderate active groups had higher mean scores and higher percentages with good scores on the MMSE than the low active group. For example, at follow-up six of the high active group had a mean score of 26.3 versus 24.9 for the low active group. While a difference of 1.4 may seem negligible on a scale of 30, most of the variation on the MMSE in the unimpaired occurs between about 22 and 30. About 80% of the moderate and high active achieved a good score versus 70% of the low active.

Table 5.2 presents the association between cognitive function and basic demographic and health characteristics. The physically capable consist of participants who reported they did not need help to do heavy work around the house, walk one half

Table 5.2 – Crude association between physical activity and cognitive function: New Haven EPESE

Level of physical activity	Number	Mean MMSE[1] score	Percent with good cognitive function[2]
Gender			
Male	463	26.2**	79.5
Female	763	25.5***	75.6***
Age			
65–74	860	26.2***	80.3***
75–84	325	25.0***	71.4**
85+	41	23.7	53.7
Education			
High school or greater	427	27.6***	92.7***
Less than high school	799	24.8	68.7
Depressive sympyoms			
Low (CESD <16)	1004	26.1***	79.3***
High (CESD ≥16)	222	24.8	67.1
Physically capable			
Yes	581	26.6***	83.5***
No	645	25.1	71.3
Self-rated health			
Good to excellent	729	26.4***	80.9***
Fair to bad	497	25.0	71.4

[1] Mini-Mental State Examination
[2] Score 24 to 30 on MMSE
**p<0.01; ***p<0.001

mile or climb a flight of stairs. Men, those aged 65-74 years at study entry, those with a high school education, those with low depressive symptoms, those with good physical function and those with good to excellent self-rated health have significantly higher mean MMSE scores than their counterparts. With the exception of men, all of these groups have higher percentages with good scores, as well. Some of the group differences are sizable – age and education, for instance.

Table 5.3 shows the association between physical activity and the same demographic and health characteristics presented in Table 5.2. All of these factors are also significantly associated with activity level. The highly and moderately active are younger on average, are more likely to be male, have lower rates of high depressive symptomatology, are more likely to be physically capable, and are more likely to have good to excellent health than those with very low or no activity. The highly active also have much higher rate of high school education – 50% versus 30%.

The associations presented in Tables 5.2 and 5.3 clearly show that the observed relationship between physical activity and cognitive performance may be, in large part, spurious, that is merely a function of the independent relationship of each of these qualities to a variety of social, demographic and health factors. Thus an important question to address is, after accounting for the differences in demographic and health characteristics between the activity groups, does the association between cognitive function and physical activity remain?

For the next set of analyses, the moderate and high active groups were combined as they share many of the same characteristics. Table 5.4 compares crude and adjusted mean MMSE scores and the percentages with good scores of low actives with moderate to high actives. The first column shows the crude associations, the second column, labeled model 1, gives the scores and percentages adjusted for age and education, model 2 adjusts for depressive symptoms, physical capability, and self-rated health, and model 3 adjusts for all five covariates. Accounting for differences in

Table 5.3 – *Association between physical activity and correlates of cognitive function*

	Level of physical activity		
	Low	**Moderate**	**High**
Mean age			
Male	73.0	71.8**	71.3***
Female	27.6	45.9***	49.8***
65-74	31.2	29.6	50.2***
75-84	26.1	9.7***	11.4***
85+	29.6	65.4***	63.5***
High school or greater	48.5	69.8***	70.3***

**p<0.01; ***p<0.001

Table 5.4 – Crude and adjusted associations between physicals activity and cognitive function

Level of physical activity	Mean MMSE[1]			
	Crude	Model1	Model 2	Model 3
Level of physical activity				
Moderate	73.0	71.8**		71.3***
Moderate	27.6	45.9***		49.8***

Level of physical activity	Percent with good score[2]			
	Crude	Model1	Model 2	Model 3
Level of physical activity				
Moderate	31.2	29.6		50.2***
Moderate	26.1	9.7***		11.4***

1 Mini-Mental State Examination
2 Score 24 to 30 on MMSE
**p<0.01; ***p<0.001; p= probability of a difference between high or moderate activity versus low.
Model 1 adjusts for age, education; Model 2 adjusts for depressive symptoms, self-rate health disability;
Model 3 adjusts for all covariates.

age and education reduces group differences but does not eliminate them. The moderate to high actives continue to perform better than the low actives. Accounting for differences in the health–related factors however, obliterates group differences. Do these findings demonstrate that physical activity has no real effect on cognitive function? Not necessarily. If physical activity influences cognition through its impact on health (recall the discussion of indirect mechanisms above), a reduction in the strength of the association between physical activity and cognitive performance is exactly what should be expected. Because the analyses are cross-sectional, the direction of influence between physical activity and health, for instance, cannot be determined.

Longitudinal analyses were conducted that examined change in MMSE score over a 3-year period for four activity groups - chronic inactive, new inactive, new active, and chronic active. The chronic inactive consisted of those classified as inactive at both the third and sixth follow-ups, the new inactive consisted of those active at the third follow-up and inactive at the sixth, the new active were inactive at the third and active at the sixth follow-up, and the chronic active consisted of those active at both follow-ups. Table 5.5 presents mean change in MMSE score for each of the four groups, unadjusted and adjusted for three different sets of factors. Model 1 adjusts for follow-up three MMSE score; model 2 adjusts for follow-up three MMSE score and age, education and gender; and model 3 adjusts for model 2 factors and interim stroke and myocardial infarction. The reference group for all comparisons is the new active. A positive change score indicates decline and a negative score, improvement.

Table 5.5 – Longitudinal association between physical activity and cognitive decline

Physical activity profile	Number	Mean change in MMSE score[1]			
		Crude	Model 1	Model 2	Model 3
1. Inactive F3 and F6	383	0.17***	0.26***	0.26***	0.26***
2. Active F3, inactive F6	219	0.37***	0.37***	0.34***	0.33***
3. Inactive F3, ActiveF6	172	-0.23	-0.18	-0.22	-0.22
4. Active F3 and F6	452	0.17***	0.08	0.16*	0.17**

1 MMSE = Mini-Mental State Examination; Change= Follow 3 score minus Follow 6 score.
p = probability of group mean change different from group 3; *p<0.05; **p<0.01; p<0.001;
Model 1 adjusts for F3 MMSE score; Model 2 adjusts for F3 MMSE score, age, education, and gender;
Model 3 adjusts for F3 MMSE score, age, education, gender, and interim stroke and myocardial infarction.

All groups experienced a decline in MMSE score over the 3-year period, except for the new active, those who were inactive at follow-up three and active at follow-up six. This association supports a positive role for physical activity. The advantage of the new active relative to the chronic active was unexpected as was the lack of advantage of the chronic active over the chronic inactive – all of these observations warrent further exploration. Those who became inactive experienced the greatest decline in MMSE score. Adjusting for initial score, the chronically active and new active appear more similar. However, adjusting for demographic factors and interim severe health events as well does not radically change the findings. Whether change in activity conditioned the change in cognitive function or whether a decline or improvement in health status, for instance, contributed to both activity level at follow-up six and performance on the MMSE remains unknown.

The analysis findings reported above should not be considered definitive, but rather illustrative of the methodologic difficulties inherent in epidemiologic investigations of the relationship between physical activity and cognitive function.

CONCLUSION

Physical activity and cognitive function are clearly associated. In persons at risk, a large majority of the older population, physical activity appears to be effective for primary and secondary prevention of cognitive decline associated with a variety of health conditions. The physical health benefits of regular exercise are well-documented and in so far as physical health influences cognitive function, physical activity should as well. In relatively healthy older persons, findings from well-controlled experiments suggest that physical activity may contribute to the maintenance of and possible improvement in the processing speed component of cognitive function.

RESEARCH RECOMMENDATIONS

Much remains unknown about the relationship between physical activity and cognitive function.[42] Three types of studies that would greatly enhance and contribute further to our understanding of this relationship include:

1. Well-controlled longitudinal observational studies. The longitudinal analysis using the New Haven EPESE data is one of the few investigations of the relationship between physical activity and cognitive function over time.

2. Long-term large sample well-controlled experiments and intervention trials. Many of the existing experimental studies have serious limitations in terms of both the number of subjects involved and the nature and duration of the exercise regimen. The FICSIT trials[43] and subsequent studies supported by the National Institute on Aging provide a good model for this effort.

3. Studies directed at identifying effective behavioral change strategies for older adults. These can and should be incorporated into the experimental studies, both in the design of the interventions and analysis plans. Few adults get adequate physical activity; promoting the adoption of regular exercise may present the greatest challenge.

REFERENCES

1. Christensen H, Mackinnon A. The association between mental, social, and physical activity and cognitive performance in young and old subjects. *Age Aging* 1993; **22**: 175-182.

2. Clarkson-Smith L, Hartley AA. Relationships between physical exercise and cognitive abilities in older adults. *Psychol Aging* 1989; **4(2)**: 183-189.

3. Spirduso WW. Reaction and movement time as a function of age and physical activity level. *J Gerontol* 1975; **30(4)**: 435-440.

4. Stones MJ, Kozma A. Age, exercise, and coding performance. *Psychol Aging* 1989; **4(2)**:190-194.

5. Farmer ME, White L, Kittner SJ et al. Neuropsychological test performance in Framingham: A descriptive study. *Psychol Rep* 1987; **60**: 1023-1040.

6. Scherr PA, Albert MS, Funkenstein HH et al. Correlates of cognitive function in an elderly community population. *Am J Epidemiol* 1988; **128(5)**: 1084-1101.

7. Wiederholt WC, Cahn D, Butters NM, Salmon DP, Kritz-Silverstein D, Barrett-Connor E. Effects of age, gender and education on selected neuropsychological tests in an elderly community cohort. *J Am Geriatr Soc* 1993; **41**: 639-647.

8. Dishman RK. Determinants of physical activity and exercise for persons 65 years of age or older. In: Spirduso WW, Eckert ?? (eds) *Physical Activity and Aging*, 1989, pp 140-162.

9. Mangione CM, Seddon JM, Cook EF et al. Correlates of cognitive function scores in elderly out patients. *J Am Geriatr Soc* 1993; **41**: 491-497.

10. Sallis JF, Haskell WL, Wood PD et al. Physical activity assessment methodology in the five-city project. *Am J Epidemiol* 1985; **121(1)**: 91-106.

11. Simonsick EM, Lafferty ME, Phillips CL *et al.* Risk due to inactivity in physically capable older adults. *Am J Public Health* 1993; **83:** 1443-1450.

12. Milligan WL, Powell DA, Harley C, Furchtgott E. A comparison of physical health and psychosocial variables as predictors of reaction time and serial learning. *J Gerontol* 1984; **39(6):** 704-710.

13. Perlmutter M, Nyquist L. Relationships between self-reported physical and mental health and intelligence performance across adulthood. *J Gerontol* 1990; **45(4):** P145-P155.

14. Lichtenberg PA, Ross T, Millis SR, Manning CA. The relationship between depression and cognition in older adults: A cross-validation study. *J Gerontol* 1995; **50B:** P25-P22.

15. King DA, Caine ED, Conwell Y, Cox C. The neuropsychology of depression in the elderly: A comparative study of normal aging and Alzeimer's disease. *J Neuropsychiat Clin Neurosci* 1991; **3:** 64-66.

16. Williams JM, Little MM, Scates S, Blockman N. Memory complaints and abilities among depressed older adults. *J Clin Consult Psychol* 1987; **55:** 595-598.

17. Farmer ME, Locke BZ, Moscicki EK, Dannenberg AL, Larson DB, Radloff LS. Physical activity and depressive symptoms: The NHANES I Epidemiologic Follow-Up Study. *Am J Epidemiol* 1988; **128(6):** 1340-1351.

18. Frederick T, Frerichs RR, Clark VA. Personal health habits and symptoms of depression at the community level. *Prev Med* 1988; **17:** 173-182.

19. Simonsick EM. Personal health habits and mental health in a national probability sample. *Am J Prev Med* 1991; **7(6):** 425-437.

20. McMahon M, Palmer R. Exercise and hypertension. *Med Clin North Am* 1985; **69(1):** 57-69.

21. Tipton CM. Exercise, training and hypertension. *Exer Sport Sci Rev* 1984; **12:** 245-306.

22. Gifford RW. Geriatric hypertension: Chairmen's comments on the NIH Working Group report. *Geriatrics* 1987; **42:** 45-50.

23. King AC, Tribble DL. The role of exercise in weight regulation in nonathletes. *Sports Med* 1991; **11(5):** 331-349.

24. Bray GA. Pathophysiology of obesity. *Am J Clin Nutr* 1992; **55:** 488S-494S.

25. Campbell AJ, Busby WJ, Horwath CC, Robertson MC. Relation of age, exercise, anthropometric measurements, and diet with glucose and insulin levels in a population aged 70 years and older. *Am J Epidemiol* 1993; **138(9):** 688-696.

26. Hachinski V. Preventable senility: a call for action against the vascular dementias. *Lancet* 1992; **340:** 645-648.

27. King AC, Taylor CB, Haskell W. Effects of differing intensities and formats of 12 months of exercise training on psychological outcomes in older adults. *Health Psychol* 1993; **12(4):** 292-300.

28. Dustman RE, Ruhling RO, Russell EM *et al.* Aerobic exercise training and improved neuropsychological function of older individuals. *Neurobiol Aging* 1984; **5:** 35-42.

29. Rogers RL, Meyer JS, Mortel KF. After reaching retirement age physical activity sustains cerebral perfusion and cognition. *J Am Geriatr Soc* 1990; **38:** 123-128.

30. Barry AJ, Steinmetz JR, Page HF, Rodahl K. The effects of physical conditioning on older individuals. II. Motor performance and cognitive function. *J Gerontol* 1966; **21:** 192-199.

31. Blumenthal JA, Emery CF, Madden DJ et al. Long-term effects of exercise on psychological functioning in older men and women. *J Gerontol* 1991; **46(6):** P352-P361.

32. Elsayed M, Ismail AH, Young RJ. Intellectual differences of adult men related to age and physical fitness before and after an exercise program. *J Gerontol* 1980; **35(3):** 383-387.

33. Emery CF, Blumenthal JA. Effects of physical exercise on psychological and cognitive functioning of older adults. *Ann Behav Med* 1991; **13(3):** 99-107.

34. Emery CF, Gatz M. Psychological and cogntive effects of an exercise program for community-residing older adults. *Gerontologist* 1990; **30(2):** 184-188.

35. Madden DJ, Blumenthal JA, Allen PA, Emery CF. Improving aerobic capacity in healthy older adults does not necessarily lead to improved cognitive performance. *Psychol Aging* 1989; **4(3):** 307-320.

36. Perri S, Templer DI. The effects of an aerobic exercise program on psychological variables in older adults. *Int J Aging Human Dev* 1984-85; **20(3):** 167-172.

37. Rikili RE, Edwards DJ. Effects of a three-year exercise program on motor function and cognitive processing speed in older women. *Res Q Exer Sport* 1991; **62(1):** 61-67.

38. Cornoni-Huntley J, Ostfeld AM, Taylor JO et al. Established populations for epidemiologic studies of the elderly: Study design and methodology. *Aging Clin Exp Res* 1993; **5:** 27-37.

39. Folstein MF, Folstein SE, McHugh PR. 'Mini-Mental State'. A practical method for grading the cognitive state of patients for the clinician. *J Psychiatr Res* 1975; **12:** 189-98.

40. Tombaugh TN, McIntyre NJ. The Mini-Mental State Examination: A comprehensive review. *J Am Geriatr Soc* 1992; **40:** 922-35.

41. Radloff LS. The CES-D scale: A self-report depression scale for research in the general population. *Appl Psychol Measurement* 1975; **1:** 385-401.

42. Buchner DM, Beresford SAA, Larson EB, LaCroix AZ, Wagner EH. Effects of physical activity on health status in older adults II: Intervention studies. *Annu Rev Pub Health* 1992; **13:** 469-488.

43. Ory MG, Schechtman KB, Miller JP et al. Fraility and injuries in later life: The FICSIT trials. *J Am Geriatr Soc* 1993; **41(3):** 283-296.

6

VASCULAR FACTORS IN COGNITIVE DECLINE

Raymond T.F. Cheung and Vladimir Hachinski

Developmental neurobiology reminds us that everyone is born with the maximal number of neurons, and that dying neurons are not replaced. Accordingly, studies show a steady decline in cerebral blood flow and metabolism with advancing age that have no direct or simple relationship with cognitive decline.[1,2] While age-related cognitive decline is almost universal, preventable or modifiable factors are probably involved, as the rate of cognitive decline is highly individual.

Dementia is an acquired condition of chronic global cognitive decline sufficiently severe to interfere with an independent social or occupational existence. Three broad etiological groups of dementia exist, including primary degenerative dementia such as Alzheimer's disease, vascular dementia, and other dementia. As vascular dementia and some other types of dementia have risk factors amenable to treatment and prevention, it becomes important to identify impaired cognitive functions from very mild to very severe. Efforts and attention should be directed to modifiable factors in aged populations at all stages of cognitive decline before dementia is established.[3]

As longevity becomes common, the proportion of the elderly in the general population is rising in most parts of the world.[4] As both cognitive decline and dementia occur more frequently with advancing age, cognitive decline of varying severity is one of the greatest problems for mankind.

VASCULAR COGNITIVE IMPAIRMENT

Definition

The concept of vascular cognitive impairment has been recently introduced with emphasis on the potential pathogenic role of vascular mechanisms in causing cognitive impairment of any severity and on the importance of early intervention.[3,5] These vascular mechanisms are ischemia, hypoxia, hemorrhage and blood–brain–barrier dysfunction. At an asymptomatic brain-at-risk stage, vascular mechanisms exist but cognition is intact; modification of risk factors is most effective in preventing cerebrovascular damage. The next pre-dementia stage encompasses a continuous spectrum of cognitive impairment short of the current definition of dementia; control of risk factors retards the rate of cognitive decline. Finally, the dementia stage sets in, and treatment becomes less effective. At present, reliable methods are not yet available to prove or disprove a causative role of vascular mechanisms in a given individual, and so coexistence by chance of a vascular mechanism (without causing cognitive impairment) or an underlying primary dementing disease cannot be recognized. On the other hand, the concept still applies when both vascular mechanisms and primary degenerative dementia contribute to cognitive impairment, because only vascular mechanisms are modifiable. Risk factors for vascular mechanisms of cognitive impairment are probably similar to those for stroke, coronary artery disease, atherosclerosis and arteriolosclerosis, and so treatment and prevention of vascular cognitive impairment are feasible.

Vascular mechanisms

The human brain, being highly complex and integrated, functions efficiently through interconnected neural networks. A variable but limited amount of cerebral damage can be tolerated without any apparent effect on cerebral functions; cognitive impairment does not occur until the total extent of cerebral damage exceeds certain threshold levels. Thus, all vascular mechanisms for cerebral damage should be detected early and treated appropriately. These vascular mechanisms are grouped into:

1. cerebral infarcts;

2. white matter damage;

3. intracranial hemorrhages;

4. blood–brain–barrier dysfunction;

5. cerebrovascular dysautoregulation and hemodynamic mechanisms.

More often than not, several vascular mechanisms exert their effects, both independently and interactively with one another, synergistically or multiplicatively to cause more damage. In addition, there are substantial overlaps among risk factors for various vascular mechanisms.

Cerebral infarcts

Stroke is one of the most important causes of morbidity and mortality, and the most common subtype is ischemic cerebral infarction. In addition to focal neurological deficits, extensive and/or multiple strokes impair cognitive function. In a prospective 4-year follow-up study,[6] 5 of 37 patients, who had cerebral infarction and normal intellectual functions initially, developed progressive intellectual deterioration at 1-4 years after stroke; 3 fulfilled the criteria for dementia (according to the Diagnostic and Statistical Manual of Mental Disorders, third edition, 1980) and multi-infarct dementia[7] (according to Hachinski's ischemic score[8]), whereas 2 had significant but milder intellectual impairment. In addition, 4 of these 5 patients had, on computed tomography of the head, multiple, bilateral cerebral infarcts when the intellectual impairment was diagnosed, despite the lack of a history of recurrent stroke.

Prevalence of dementia and incidence of new-onset dementia (according to the examining neurologist's best judgement) among survivors of acute ischemic stroke in the Stroke Data Bank cohort have been recently reported.[9] One hundred and sixteen (16%) of 726 testable patients were regarded as demented when examined within 10 days of stroke onset; prevalence was related to age, previous stroke, and previous myocardial infarction. Number and location of infarcts and presence of cortical atrophy on computed tomography of the head were also associated with prevalence of dementia. Kaplan-Meier analysis of incidence of new-onset dementia during a 2-year follow-up among the remaining 610 patients, who were not demented initially, showed the effects of age; the chance of new-onset dementia at 1 year was 5.4% for patients 60 years of age and 10.4% for patients aged 90.[9]

As these two studies[6,9] focused on major impairment in cognitive functions, milder degrees of cognitive impairment after stroke could be a common problem. Nevertheless, a significant number of these patients might have coexisting primary degenerative dementia with varying contributions to the cognitive impairment.

Volume, bilaterality, location, and number of cerebral infarcts are important determinants for cognitive impairment after stroke.[9-12] In a classical pathological study of 50 demented patients and 28 non-demented controls,[13] the total volume of infarction was associated with dementia. Only 2 of the 28 controls had more than 50 ml of cerebral softening whereas 16 of the 50 demented patients had more than this volume, and all 9 cases with more than 100 ml of cerebral softening had dementia. Nevertheless, more recent clinical-radiological[14] or clinical-pathological[15] study indicates that most patients with vascular dementia have less than 100 ml of brain infarction. In addition, bilateral infarcts are more common than unilateral infarcts in vascular dementia.[9,11,12] Bilaterality is important probably because of the bilateral location of brain structures subserving memory function and because of a larger total volume of infarcts. The concept of strategic-infarct dementia illustrates the importance of location.[10,16,17] Infarction of the angular gyrus in the dominant hemisphere, paramedial thalamus (especially bilateral) or head of caudate nucleus can cause major cognitive and neuropsychological impairment. The number of infarcts is probably not an independent factor but relates to the other factors.[12] For example, multiple lacunar infarcts are associated with cognitive impairment.[18]

Immediate pathogenic mechanisms for cerebral infarcts of various sizes are artery-to-artery embolism, thrombosis of an extracranial or intracranial artery, cardiogenic embolism, lacunar infarction and small vessel disease, hypoperfusion of the brain (causing watershed infarcts), hemorrheological (hyperviscosity) factors, hypercoagulability, inflammatory and non-inflammatory (amyloid angiopathy) cerebral arteriopathies, and hereditary vascular diseases.

White matter damage

Destruction or demyelination of white matter causes disconnection and functional deficits;[19] its role in vascular cognitive impairment resembles cerebral infarcts in gray matter. Advances in neuroimaging have caused an epidemic of 'Binswanger's disease' which is 'neither Binswanger's nor a disease'.[20] Widespread white matter changes occur in vascular dementia, Alzheimer's disease, demyelinating disorders and even normal aging.[21]

Reduced attenuation of white matter or leukoaraiosis[22] in computed tomography of the head has been related pathologically to partial loss of myelin, axons and oligodendrocytes, diffuse demyelination, reactive astrocytic gliosis, small infarcts, arteriolar sclerosis, dilatation of the ventricular system or perivascular spaces, and vascular ectasia.[1,23] Leukoaraiosis appears as white matter hyperintensity on T2-weighted magnetic resonance imaging of the head. A recent magnetic resonance imaging and pathological study of lesions in the centrum ovale of 15 unselected autopsies revealed two types of hyperintensity on magnetic resonance imaging: extensive and punctate.[24] Extensive hyperintensities correspond pathologically to areas of loss of axons, myelin, and oligodendrocytes, with spongiosis but not infarction. Punctate hyperintensities are less well defined but commonly relate to dilated perivascular spaces. The presence of leukoaraiosis is associated with advancing age, deteriorating intellectual functions, hypertension, stroke, gait disturbance, unprovoked fall, cardiovascular disease, and diabetes mellitus.[21,25-29]

Immediate pathogenic mechanisms for ischemic white matter changes are the same as those for cerebral infarction, but small vessel disease, cerebral hypoperfusion, inflammatory and non-inflammatory cerebral arteriopathies are more important. Pathogenic mechanisms for non-ischemic white matter changes are diverse and related to the underlying pathologies. The latter include demyelination, defective myelination, inflammation, infection, and edema.

Intracranial hemorrhages

Intracranial hemorrhage such as intracerebral hemorrhage, subarachnoid hemorrhage, subdural hematoma, or extradural hematoma, produces widespread cerebral destruction, increases intracranial pressure, and compresses nearby structures. Multiple intracerebral hemorrhages with or without obstructive hydrocephalus or subdural hematoma often cause major cognitive decline.[30] Hypertension, cerebral amyloid angiopathy, and trauma are the most important risk factors.

Blood-brain-barrier dysfunction

Analyses of cerebrospinal fluid reveal an elevated albumin level or ratio (of cerebrospinal fluid protein level to plasma protein level) in patients with vascular dementia or Alzheimer's disease, suggesting blood-brain-barrier deficiency.[31-33] In addition, cerebrospinal fluid protein abnormalities are associated with leukoaraiosis.[34] The underlying mechanism is probably a persistent vessel wall disturbance. Risk factors for blood-brain-barrier dysfunction are largely unknown, but small vessel disease may be a major factor.

Cerebrovascular dysautoregulation and hemodynamic mechanisms

Normal fluctuations in blood pressure with diurnal cycle, activity, and emotional changes do not cause brain damage because of the autoregulation of cerebral blood flow. Stiffening of cerebral arteries and impaired cerebrovascular autoregulation may develop from cerebral arteriolosclerosis, amyloid angiopathy, and/or non–amyloid angiopathy. Excessive antihypertensive treatment together with cerebrovascular dysautoregulation may produce cerebral damage during episodes of hypoperfusion.[21,35]

Impaired cerebrovascular autoregulation makes the brain vulnerable to hemodynamic disturbances. Systemic hypotension due to cardiovascular diseases, cerebral hypoperfusion due to a severely stenosed or occluded carotid artery, or severe hypoxia due to pulmonary disorders can cause ischemic or anoxic cerebral damage. In addition, the location of hemodynamic damage is in the vascular watershed areas such as the cerebral cortex between territories of major cerebral arteries, the basal area between the head of the caudate nucleus, internal capsule and putamen, and the periventricular white matter areas.[35]

Vascular risk factors

In general, risk factors for vascular cognitive impairment, stroke, and coronary artery disease are probably the same.[21,36] Vascular risk factors include atherosclerosis, hypertension, cardiac disease, carotid stenosis, transient ischemic attacks and stroke, cigarette smoking, abnormal lipids, obesity, diabetes mellitus, dietary factors, alcohol abuse, antiphospholipid antibody syndrome and other prothrombotic states, hemodynamic disturbances, hyperviscosity, elevated fibrinogen, cerebral amyloid angiopathy and other arteriopathy, arteriovenous malformation, and trauma. Frequently, several risk factors coexist in the same individual and interact with one another.

Artherosclerosis

Atherosclerosis of the large extracranial arteries is a major cause of ischemic stroke in caucasians. On the other hand, intracranial atherosclerosis is more important in blacks and orientals.[37] The immediate mechanism is commonly either atherothrombosis or embolism. Less frequently, hemodynamic compromise develops in the presence of very tight stenosis or total occlusion. In addition, atherosclerosis of the ascending aorta has been recently associated with embolic stroke.[38] Finally, ischemic heart disease due to coronary atherosclerosis can lead to cardiogenic cerebral emboli or cerebral hypoperfusion.

The earliest lesion of atherosclerosis is fatty streaks; these may be found in adolescence.[39] Some fatty streaks evolve into fibrous plaques of variable composition and consistency. While fibrous plaques may enlarge and compromise blood flow, complicated atheromatous plaques slowly appear, following calcium accumulation, ulceration, rupture, intraplaque hemorrhage, and reorganization. Distribution of advanced atherosclerotic plaques in the arterial tree is neither uniform nor random. Disturbed flow pattern with local shear stresses at arterial bifurcation is an important local hemodynamic factor explaining the common sites of atherosclerotic plaque formation.

Abnormal lipid patterns, hypertension, smoking, and genetic predisposition are the major risk factors for atherosclerosis. Elevated total and low-density lipoprotein cholesterol raises the risk of atherosclerosis whereas increased high-density lipoprotein cholesterol is protective.[39] The relationship between hypertension and atherosclerosis is indirect and complex, as atherosclerosis is probably a remodeling process in response to disturbances in laminar flow pattern.[40] Hypertension increases flow velocity and causes turbulence, and thus may enhance atherosclerosis from shear stresses. Homozygous homocystinuria is an autosomal recessive Mendelian disorder in which premature generalized atherosclerosis, thrombo-embolic complications, and renovascular hypertension develop in the presence of homocysteinemia.[41]

At present, treatment of extracranial and intracranial atherosclerosis involves control of risk factors (to retard the progression) and prevention of atherothromboembolic complications (by antiplatelet agents and/or carotid endarterectomy).[42] In the future, effective and specific anti-atherosclerotic agents may become available.

Hypertension
Hypertension, systolic and/or diastolic, is one of the most important risk factor for atherosclerosis, coronary artery disease, stroke (including atherothrombotic and lacunar infarction, intracerebral hemorrhage, and subarachnoid hemorrhage), and vascular dementia.[40,43,44] In addition, hypertension is associated with, on neuro-imaging, white matter changes and cerebral atrophy.[45,46] Hypertension also causes small vessel disease or arteriolosclerosis, and so cerebrovascular dysauto-regulation and blood-brain-barrier dysfunctions may occur. Finally, excessive or inappropriate treatment of hypertension produces secondary damage by causing hypoperfusion, adverse effects on lipids, electrolyte disturbances (like hypokalemia), impaired glucose tolerance, and accelerated atherosclerosis.

Acute severe hypertension leads to hypertensive encephalopathy when cerebrovascular autoregulation fails.[40] Widespread arteriolar dilatations occur with increased local cerebral blood flow, vasocongestion, and cerebral edema. Simultaneously, multifocal cerebral ischemia develops because of fibrinoid necrosis and occlusion of small arteries and arterioles. Urgent medical treatment with either continuous infusion or small, repeated intravenous doses of potent antihypertensive drugs under close monitoring should be given and overtreatment with resulting cerebral and myocardial ischemia avoided.

Concerning chronic effects, hypertension causes both tensile and shear stresses on arterial walls as well as increasing cardiac afterload. Arteriolar microaneurysms and occlusion of arterioles and small arteries are long-term effects of the tensile stress of hypertension.[40,43] Hypertensive intracerebral hemorrhages are due to rupture of arteriolar microaneurysms in the basal ganglia, thalamus, pons or cerebellum (the vascular centrencephalon). Detection and treatment of hypertension have reduced the incidence of hypertensive intracerebral hemorrhage, and consequently, multifocal, superficial, lobar hemorrhages due to cerebral amyloid angiopathy become more common.[47]

Lacunar infarctions are small infarcts in the white matter or deep gray nuclei of the vascular centrencephalon; the underlying occlusion of small arteries and arterioles is due to fibrinoid necrosis, emboli from a proximal source, and ostial obstruction from atherosclerosis. Multiple lacunes are associated with cognitive decline and leukoaraiosis.[18]

Two factors help to explain the lack of effectiveness of antihypertensive therapy in preventing atherothrombotic stroke. Adverse effects of some antihypertensive drugs on lipids may accelerate atherosclerosis. In addition, accelerated heart rate from vasodilators and/or diuretics can produce flow disturbances. There is some preliminary evidence that antihypertensive drugs like cardio-selective beta-blockers, calcium channel antagonists, and angiotensin-converting-enzyme inhibitors may have anti-atherosclerotic effects.[40]

Cardiac disease

Leukoaraiosis is associated with cardiac diseases,[28] which cause cerebral damage by producing emboli or systemic hypotension. Cardiogenic cerebral or systemic embolism, being a more common mechanism than systemic hypotension, occurs in a high number of cardiac diseases, including atrial fibrillation with or without mitral valve disease or thyrotoxicosis, ischemic heart disease with acute myocardial infarction or ventricular aneurysm, rheumatic or prosthetic valvular heart disease, infective endocarditis, mitral valve prolapse, and paradoxical embolism.[38,48] The first three are common, and treatment is anticoagulation unless otherwise contraindicated. Risk of bleeding, treatment compliance and availability of monitoring should be considered in individual patients. Although aspirin is less effective than coumadin in stroke prophylaxis in patients with non–valvular atrial fibrillation, aspirin is better than placebo.[42] Thus, aspirin is an acceptable alternative to life–long therapy with coumadin for younger patients with low risk profiles and for those in whom coumadin is unsafe. Surgical and medical therapies are also useful in some of these cardiac diseases.

Emboli may originate from a prolapsing mitral valve, but this condition is common in the general population, especially in young females. Similarly, patent foramen ovale occurs frequently in normal people. In general, the risk of embolism for these two conditions does not warrant prophylactic antithrombotic therapy for primary prevention.[49] When mitral valve prolapse and patent foramen ovale are discovered in patients with cerebrovascular ischemic symptoms, other mechanisms should be considered and the best clinical judgement made on an individual basis.[38]

Long-term anticoagulation, even within the therapeutic range, is associated with an extra 1–2% annual risk for fatal or major bleeding, including intracranial hemorrhage.[49] Septic or mycotic aneurysms of infective endocarditis are particularly prone to rupture, resulting in massive, often fatal, intracerebral bleeding.[50] Hemorrhagic infarction is associated with embolic stroke; the severity of hemorrhage varies from a few petechiae to a hematoma.[51] The proposed mechanism is diapedesis of blood through damaged small vessels, within an area of ischemic cerebral infarction, during reperfusion.

Systemic hypotension due to cardiac failure, acute myocardial infarction, or arrhythmias can cause cerebral hypoperfusion and infarctions in the watershed regions. Treatment depends on the underlying mechanisms and is largely medical.

Carotid stenosis

Extracranial carotid stenosis is an established risk factor for symptomatic and silent stroke. Nevertheless, the risk for stroke is non–uniform but affected by factors such as occurrence of symptoms, degree of stenosis, presence of ulceration, contralateral occlusion, presence of collaterals, a number of other risk factors, and cerebral infarction on computed tomography of the head.[52] Randomized clinical trials[53,54] have indicated the safety and effectiveness of elective carotid endarterectomy in patients with symptomatic carotid stenosis of 70–99% (according to the measurement used in the North American Symptomatic Carotid Endarterectomy Trial). Currently, scientific data do not unequivocally support the use of carotid endarterectomy in patients with asymptomatic stenosis and in those with milder stenosis, and so the treatment should be antithrombotic therapy and modification of risk factors.[55]

Pathologically, carotid stenosis is due to atheromatous plaques in the great majority of cases.[56] Very occasionally, fibromuscular dysplasia or other rare conditions cause the stenosis.[57] There are two immediate pathogenic mechanisms for cerebrovascular ischemic symptoms and/or signs in carotid stenosis: thromboembolic (especially with an ulcerated plaque) and hemodynamic (when there is near or total occlusion, especially with poor collaterals and/or systemic hypotension).

Transient ischemic attacks and stroke

Transient ischemic attacks and stroke are manifestations of cerebrovascular damage and risk factors for future cerebrovascular and cardiovascular events and leukoaraiosis. Assessments and investigations should disclose the underlying vascular mechanisms and risk factors so that effective treatment and prevention can be provided. As discussed above, cerebral damage, however small, may reduce the threshold for subsequent development of vascular cognitive impairment. Treatment includes antiplatelet agents, anticoagulation, carotid endarterectomy, and/or modification of risk factors.[42,58]

Cigarette smoking

Smoking is an important vascular risk factor for atherosclerosis, stroke, and cardiovascular diseases, in addition to its role in pulmonary diseases. One pathogenic mechanism of smoking is the enhancement of breakdown of elastic tissue in lungs and arteries, predisposing to saccular aneurysm formation and subarachnoid hemorrhage.[59] Theoretically, this risk factor is most amenable to modification, and cessation of smoking should be encouraged in all smokers.

Abnormal lipids

Dyslipoproteinemia is associated with premature atherosclerosis, ischemic heart disease, and ischemic stroke.[60] A high level of total and low-density lipoprotein cholesterols, a reduced level of high-density lipoprotein cholesterol, and an increased ratio of low- to high-density lipoprotein cholesterols constitute the dyslipoproteinemia. Lipoprotein a is closely related to low-density lipoprotein, but whether it is an independent risk factor for atherosclerosis or an epiphenomenon related to low-density lipoprotein is uncertain.[61] Dietary restriction, exercise, weight loss, stress management, and drug therapy are effective in improving the lipid pattern whereas high cholesterol intake, a sedentary lifestyle, and smoking worsen the pattern.

Apolipoprotein E is involved in mobilizing and redistributing cholesterol during neuronal growth and after injury and in transporting lipids through cerebrospinal fluid.[62] Recent studies have suggested that apolipoprotein E ε4 allele is a susceptibility factor and ε2 allele a protective factor for the development of Alzheimer's disease.[63,64] The facts that apolipoprotein E is associated with coronary artery disease and atherosclerosis and that Alzheimer's disease is associated with leukoaraiosis, cerebral amyloid angiopathy and blood-brain-barrier dysfunctions, suggest the presence of some treatable vascular components in Alzheimer's disease.[32,35]

Obesity

Obesity is probably not an independent factor but related to dyslipoproteinemia, increased blood pressure, glucose intolerance, dietary indiscretion, and lack of exercise. In experimental animal studies, caloric restriction prolongs survival.[4]

Diabetes mellitis

Diabetes mellitus is associated with atherosclerosis, dyslipoproteinemia, coronary artery disease, cerebrovascular disease (including small vessel disease), hypertension, obesity, and leukoaraiosis.[65]

Dietary factors

Low dietary salt intake improves hypertension. In addition, dietary restriction of cholesterol, fats, and calories is important for dyslipoproteinemia, obesity, and diabetes mellitus. A prospective 12-year follow-up study of 859 healthy subjects aged 50-79 years provided some preliminary evidence that dietary potassium may be vaso-protective; there was a 40% reduction in stroke mortality with a 10 mmol per day increase in dietary potassium.[66]

Alcohol abuse

Recent studies have clarified the role of alcohol consumption in stroke. Low levels of alcohol intake appear to reduce the risk for stroke by improving the lipid pattern.[65] Nevertheless, moderate-to-heavy drinking, especially with acute intoxication, increases the risk for ischemic and hemorrhagic strokes by hemoconcentration (producing hyperviscosity), hypertension (increasing the risk for intracranial bleeding), rebound thrombocytosis (causing a prothrombotic state), cardiac arrhythmias (generating thromboemboli or hypoperfusion), and interactions with smoking (as smoking is more frequent among heavy drinkers).

Prothrombotic states

Thrombosis with or without embolism is the most important mechanism for cerebrovascular ischemia. Under healthy conditions, clotting factors are inactive, and there are naturally occurring anticoagulants derived from the normal endothelium, including heparin, prostacyclin, tissue plasminogen activator, protein C and S, and antithrombin III.[39] The uncommon conditions of increased tendency to form clots are referred to as pro-thrombotic states, which include increased factor VIII, antithrombin III deficiency, proteins C and S deficiencies, anti-phospholipid antibodies syndrome (such as anticardiolipin antibodies and lupus anticoagulant), fibrinolytic insufficiency, antifibrinolytic therapy, thrombocytosis, platelet hyperaggregability, thrombotic thrombocytopenic purpura, haemolytic uraemic syndrome, chronic diffuse intravascular coagulopathy, paroxysmal nocturnal coagulopathy, nephrotic syndrome, pregnancy, and peripartum and postpartum states.[67] The possibility of dealing with prothrombotic conditions should be remembered and the diagnosis confirmed by appropriate laboratory investigations. Nevertheless, treatment decisions should be individualized and based on the underlying diagnosis.

Hemodynamic disturbances

As explained above, normal fluctuations in blood pressure are tolerated because of autoregulation of cerebral blood flow. Impaired cerebrovascular autoregulation and/or excessive fluctuations in blood pressure produce watershed infarction during cerebral hypoperfusion or intracerebral hemorrhage from rupture of an artery or arteriole during severe hypertension. Cerebrovascular responsiveness to changes in carbon dioxide tension is a good indicator of cerebral vasoreactivity and small vessel disease.[68] Twenty-four hour ambulatory blood pressure monitoring is useful in detecting excessive diurnal fluctuations in blood pressure.[69]

Hyperviscosity

Raised blood viscosity not only increases the shear stress to the arterial wall, arterial blood pressure, and tendency to thrombosis but also impedes micro-vascular flow.[70,71] Hyperviscosity occurs in polycythaemia, sickle cell disease, dysproteinaemia, and elevated fibrinogen level.[67] Despite the association between hyperviscosity and ischemic stroke, hemodilution (either isovolemic or hypovolemic) is ineffective in acute stroke therapy.[70]

Cerebral amyloid angiopathy and other arteriopathy

In cerebral amyloid angiopathy, there is infiltration of leptomeningeal and cortical penetrating arteries with amyloid; arteries in the subcortical regions and the systemic vasculature are spared.[47] Although the most common manifestation is multifocal lobar intracerebral hemorrhage, cerebral amyloid angiopathy has also been associated with normal aging, Alzheimer's disease, cerebral infarction, leukoaraiosis, seizures and subarachnoid hemorrhage. Thus, cognitive impairment or dementia develops after recurrent, multifocal ischemic and hemorrhagic cerebral damage. Hereditary cerebral hemorrhage with amyloid deposition in the brain (HCHWA) has been reported in both Icelandic (HCHWA-I)[72] and Dutch (HCHWA-D)[73] families. In both HCHWA-I and HCHWA-D, dementia occurs in up to 75% of affected individuals during the course of their illness and is sometimes the presenting problem.[72,73] The amyloid protein in HCHWA-I characteristically contains cystatin C protein,[72] whereas a mutation of the amyloid precursor protein gene on chromosome 21 is responsible for HCHWA-D.[74] Appropriate treatment for cerebral amyloid angiopathy depends on the manifestation, and antithrombotic therapy is contraindicated.

In cerebral autosomal dominant arteriopathy with subcortical infarcts and leukoen-cephalopathy (CADASIL), the causative gene has been recently localized to chromosome 19q12.[75] CADASIL presents with recurrent stroke and transient ischemic attacks, progressive pseudobulbar palsy, cerebellar signs and subcortical dementia.[76] Small arteries of the white matter and basal ganglia, and occasionally the small leptomeningeal arteries, have an extensive deposition of a granular, non-fibrinoid, eosinophilic material in the media together with frequent frag-mentation and/or reduplication of the internal elastic lamella.[76,77] Thus, CADASIL is an hereditary non-inflammatory non-amyloid cerebral angiopathy.

Arteriovenous malformation

The concept of hypoperfusion dementia secondary to cerebral arteriosclerosis prevailed in the early twentieth century, but there is little evidence for chronic ischemia.[78,79] Nevertheless, patients with mental decline due to dural arteriovenous fistula have been reported. One recent report also documented objective intellectual improvement after embolization to the fistula.[80] In general, arteriovenous malformation can occur spontaneously or after trauma or dural sinus thrombosis. Pathogenic mechanisms are arterial steal, increased venous pressure, and rupture with bleeding. Effective treatment includes surgical excision or embolization.

Miscellaneous

Trauma is associated with extradural and subdural hematoma. Direct trauma to neck arteries or chiropractic manipulation of neck is associated with arterial dissection and stroke.[81] Diffuse axonal injury after a motor vehicle accident can produce cognitive decline and memory disturbances. Abuse of drugs like amphetamine, cocaine, and heroin is associated with increased risk for intracerebral hemorrhage and cerebral infarction.[82] The underlying mechanisms appear to include allergic arteritis and sudden severe hypertension. Intravenous drug abusers are also at risk for systemic and pulmonary emboli and infection (including infective endocarditis). Heterozygous homocystinuria has been suggested to cause premature atherosclerosis and stroke.[41] Migraine is a common condition and occurrence of stroke may be coincidental.[65] Nevertheless, there is some evidence that migraineurs taking birth control pills have an increased risk for stroke. The relationship between the birth control pill per se and stroke remains controversial.[83] There is no good evidence that hyperuricemia is associated with a higher risk for stroke.[65]

CONCLUSION

There is persisting controversy about the definition of vascular dementia, the role of vascular brain damage in dementia, and the antemortem differentiation between vascular and primary degenerative dementias.[84] However, the time is ripe to discard the obsolete concept of vascular dementia; "vascular is too generic and dementia too late".[5] Recent advances in research on atherosclerosis, stroke, and coronary artery disease have paved the ground for rational, proven, effective treatment of many vascular risk factors, which produce cognitive impairment via vascular mechanisms. Human populations are aging,[4] and so cognitive decline is of increasing importance. Adopting the alternative approach under the concept of vascular cognitive impairment would permit early intervention and opportunities for longitudinal follow-up studies. The future is very promising. There is some preliminary evidence that control of blood pressure in hypertensive patients and cessation of smoking in smokers improve cognitive functions[85] and that daily use of aspirin improves cerebral perfusion and cognitive performance.[86] These are only the beginnings of the prevention and treatment of vascular cognitive impairment.

ACKNOWLEDGEMENT

V.H. is a Career Investigator of the Heart and Stroke Foundation of Canada. R.T.F.C. is a recipient of a Research Fellowship from the Medical Council of Canada.

REFERENCES

1. Kety SS. Human cerebral blood flow and oxygen consumption as related to aging. *J Chron Dis* 1956; **3**: 478-486.

2. Davis SM, Ackerman RH, Correia JA *et al.* Cerebral blood flow and cerebrovascular CO_2 reactivity in stroke-age normal controls. *Neurology* 1983; **33**: 391-399.

3. Hachinski V. Preventable senility: a call for action against the vascular dementias. *Lancet* 1992; **340**: 645-648.

4. Olshansky SJ, Carnes BA, Cassel CK. The aging of the human species. *Sci Am* 1993; **268(4)**: 46-52.

5. Hachinski V. Vascular dementia: a radical redefinition. *Dementia* 1994; **5**: 130-132.

6. Kotila M, Waltimo O, Niemi ML, Laaksonen R. Dementia after stroke. *Eur Neurol* 1986; **25**: 134-140.

7. Hachinski VC, Lassen NA, Marshall J. Multi-infarct dementia. A cause of mental deterioration in the elderly. *Lancet* 1974; **2**: 207-210.

8. Hachinski VC, Iliff LD, Zilhka E *et al.* Cerebral blood flow in dementia. *Arch Neurol* 1975; **32**: 632-637.

9. Tatemichi TK, Foulkes MA, Mohr JP *et al.* Dementia in stroke survivors in the Stroke Data Bank cohort - prevalence, incidence, risk factors, and computed tomographic findings. *Stroke* 1990; **21**: 858-866.

10. Tatemichi TK. How acute brain failure becomes chronic - a view of the mechanisms of dementia related to stroke. *Neurology* 1990; **40**: 1652-1659.

11. Tatemichi TK, Desmond DW, Paik M *et al.* Clinical determinants of dementia related to stroke. *Ann Neurol* 1993; **33**: 568-575.

12. O'Brien MD. How does cerebrovascular disease cause dementia? *Dementia* 1994: **5**: 133-136.

13. Tomlinson BE, Blessed G, Roth M. Observations on the brains of demented old people. *J Neurol Sci* 1970; **11**: 205-242.

14. Loeb C, Gandolfo C, Bino G. Intellectual impairment and cerebral lesions in multiple cerebral infarcts. A clinical-computed tomography study. *Stroke* 1988; **19**: 560-565.

15. de Ser T, Bermejo F, Portera A, Arredondo JM, Bouras C, Constantinidis J. Vascular dementia. A clinicopathological study. *J Neurol Sci* 1990; **96**: 1-17.

16. Roman GC, Tatemichi TK, Erkinjuntti T *et al.* Vascular dementia: diagnostic criteria for research studies - report of the NINDS-AIREN International Workshop. *Neurology* 1993; **43**: 250-260.

17. Garcia JH, Brown GG. Vascular dementia: neuropathologic alterations and metabolic brain changes. *J Neurol Sci* 1992; **109**: 121-131.

18. Loeb C. Dementia due to lacunar infarctions: a misnomer or a clinical entity? *Eur Neurol* 1995; **35:** 187-192.

19. Yao H, Sadoshima S, Kuwabara Y, Ichiya Y, Fujishima M. Cerebral blood flow and oxygen metabolism in patients with vascular dementia of the Binswanger type. *Stroke* 1990; **21:** 1694-1699.

20. Hachinski V. Binswanger's disease: neither Binswanger's nor a disease. *J Neurol Sci* 1991;**103:** 1.

21. Erkinjuntti T, Hachinski VC. Rethinking vascular dementia. *Cerebrovasc Dis* 1993; **3:** 3-23.

22. Hachinski VC, Potter P, Merskey H. Leuko-Araiosis. *Arch Neurol* 1987; **44:** 21-23.

23. Yamanouchi H. Loss of white matter oligodendrocytes and astrocytes in progressive subcortical vascular encephalopathy of Binswanger type. *Acta Neurol Scand* 1991; **83:** 301-305.

24. Munoz DG, Hastak SM, Harper B, Lee D, Hachinski VC. Pathologic correlates of increased signals of the centrum ovale on magnetic resonance imaging. *Arch Neurol* 1993; **50:** 492-497.

25. Steingart A, Hachinski VC, Lau C *et al*. Cognitive and neurologic findings in subjects with diffuse white matter lucencies on computed tomographic scan (Leuko-Araiosis). *Arch Neurol* 1987; **44:** 32-35.

26. Steingart A, Hachinski VC, Lau C *et al*. Cognitive and neurologic findings in demented patients with diffuse white matter lucencies on computed tomographic scan (Leuko-Araiosis). *Arch Neurol* 1987; **44:** 36-39.

27. Inzitari D, Diaz F, Fox A *et al*. Vascular risk factors and Leuko-Araiosis. *Arch Neurol* 1987; **44:** 42-47.

28. Raiha I, Tarvonen S, Kurki T, Rajala T, Sourander L. Relationship between vascular factors and white matter low attenuation of the brain. *Acta Neurol Scand* 1993; **87:** 286-289.

29. Mineura K, Sasajima H, Kikuchi K *et al*. White matter hyperintensity in neurologically asymptomatic subjects. *Acta Neurol Scand* 1995; **92:** 151-156.

30. Cummings JL. Treatable dementias. In: Mayeux R, Rosen WG (eds) *The Dementias*. Raven Press, New York, 1983, pp 165-183.

31. Mecocci P, Parnetti L, Reboldi GP *et al*. Blood-brain-barrier in a geriatric population: barrier function in degenerative and vascular dementias. *Acta Neurol Scand* 1991; **84:** 210-213.

32. Mattila KM, Pirttila T, Blennow K, Wallin A, Viitanen M, Frey H. Altered blood-brain-barrier function in Alzheimer's disease. *Acta Neurol Scand* 1994; **89:** 192-198.

33. Wallin A, Blennow K, Fredman P, Gottfries CG, Karlsson I, Svennerholm L. Blood brain barrier function in vascular dementia. *Acta Neurol Scand* 1990; **81:** 318-322.

34. Pantoni L, Inzitari D, Pracucci G et al. Cerebrospinal fluid proteins in patients with leucoaraiosis: possible abnormalities in blood-brain barrier function. *J Neurol Sci* 1993; **115:** 125-131.

35. Hachinski VC. The decline and resurgence of vascular dementia. *Can Med Assoc J* 1990; **142:** 107-111.

36. Gorelick PB, Mangone CA. Vascular dementias in the elderly. *Clin Geriatr Med* 1991; **7:** 599-615.

37. Gorelick PB. Distribution of atherosclerotic cerebrovascular lesions - effects of age, race, and sex. *Stroke* 1993; **24[suppl I]:** I-16-I-19.

38. Hart RG. Cardiogenic embolism to the brain. *Lancet* 1992; **339:** 589-594.

39. Fisher M. Cellular basis of atherosclerosis. In: Norris JW, Hachinski VC (eds) *Prevention of Stroke*. Springer-Verlag, New York, 1991 pp 19-36.

40. Spence JD, Hypertension and stroke prevention. In: Norris JW, Hachinski VC (eds). *Prevention of Stroke*. Springer-Verlag, New York, 1991, pp 113–120.

41. Boers GHJ, Smals AGH, Trijbels FJM *et al*. Heterozygosity for homocystinuria in premature peripheral and cerebral occlusive arterial disease. *N Engl J Med* 1985; **313**: 709–715.

42. Barnett HJM, Eliasziw M, Meldrum HE. Drugs and surgery in the prevention of ischemic stroke. *N Engl J Med* 1995; **332**: 238–248.

43. Phillips SJ. Pathogenesis, diagnosis, and treatment of hypertension–associated stroke. *Am J Hypertens* 1989; **2**: 493–501.

44. Forette F, Boller F. Hypertension and the risk of dementia in the elderly. *Am J Med* 1991; **90[suppl 3A]**: 14S–19S.

45. Salerno JA, Murphy DGM, Horwitz B *et al*. Brain atrophy in hypertension - a volumetric magnetic resonance imaging study. *Hypertension* 1992; **20**: 340–348.

46. Yao H, Sadoshima S, Ibayashi S, Kuwabara Y, Ichiya Y, Fujishima M. Leukoaraiosis and dementia in hypertensive patients. *Stroke* 1992; **23**: 1673–1677.

47. Feldmann E, Tornabene J. Diagnosis and treatment of cerebral amyloid angiopathy. *Clin Geriatr Med* 1995; **7**: 617–630.

48. Davis PH, Hachinski VC. The cardiac factor in stroke. *Curr Opin Neurol Neurosurg* 1992; **5**: 39–43.

49. Easton JD. Present status of anticoagulant prophylaxis. In: Norris JW, Hachinski VC (eds) *Prevention of Stroke*. Springer-Verlag, New York, 1991, pp 139–148.

50. Masuda J, Yutani C, Waki R, Ogata J, Kuriyama Y, Yamaguchi T. Histopathological analysis of the mechanisms of intracranial hemorrhage complicating infective endocarditis. *Stroke* 1992; **23**: 843–850.

51. Okada Y, Yamaguchi T, Minematsu K et al. Hemorrhagic transformation in cerebral embolism. *Stroke* 1989; **20**: 598–603.

52. Barnett HJM. Status report on the North American Symptomatic Carotid Surgery Trial. *J Mal Vasc* 1993; **18**: 202–208.

53. North American Symptomatic Carotid Endarterectomy Trial Collaborators. Beneficial effect of carotid endarterectomy in symptomatic patients with high-grade carotid stenosis. *N Engl J Med* 1991; **325**: 445–453.

54. European Carotid Surgery Trialists' Collaborative Group. MRC European Carotid Surgery Trial. interim results for symptomatic patients with severe (70-99%) or with mild (0-29%) carotid stenosis. *Lancet* 1991; **337**: 1235–1243.

55. Moore WS, Barnett HJM, Beebe HG *et al*. Guidelines for carotid endarterectomy. A multidisciplinary consensus statement from the Ad Hoc Committee, American Heart Association *Stroke* 1995; **26**: 188–201.

56. Fisher M, Martin A, Cosgrove M, Norris JW. The NASCET-ACAS plaque project. *Stroke* 1993; **24[suppl I]**: I-24-I-25.

57. Sandok BA. Fibromuscular dysplasia of the cephalic arterial system. In: Toole JF (ed) *Handbook of Clinical Neurology, Vol 11* **(55)**: Vascular Diseases, Part III. Elsevier Science Publishers, Amsterdam, 1989, pp 283–291.

58. Barnett HJM. Aspirin in stroke prevention - an overview. *Stroke* 1990; **21[suppl IV]**: IV-40-IV-43.

59. Longstreth WT, Nelson LM, Koepsell TD, van Belle G. Cigarette smoking, alcohol use and subarachnoid hemorrhage. *Stroke* 1993; **23**: 1242-1249.

60. Qizilbash N, Duffy SW, Warlow C, Mann J. Lipids are risk factors for ischaemic stroke: overview and review. *Cerebrovasc Dis* 1992; **2**: 127-136.

61. Yatsu FM, DeGraba TJ. Prevention of atherothrombotic brain infarction: role of lipids. In: Norris JW, Hachinski VC (eds) *Prevention of Stroke*. Springer-Verlag, New York, 1991, pp 37-48.

62. Harrington CR, Louwagie J, Rossau R *et al*. Influence of apolipoprotein E genotype on senile dementia of the Alzheimer and Lewy body type - significance for etiological theories of Alzheimer's disease. *Am J Path* 1994; **145**: 1472-1484.

63. Saunders AM, Strittmatter WJ, Schmechel D *et al*. Assoication of apolipoprotein E allele E4 with late-onset familial and sporadic Alzheimer's disease. *Neurology* 1993; 43: 1467-1472.

64. Frisoni GB, Calabresi L, Geroldi C et al. Apolipoprotein E e-4 allele in Alzheimer's disease and vascular dementia. *Dementia* 1994; **5**: 240-242.

65. Dyken ML. Stroke risk factors. In: Norris JW, Hachinski VC (eds). *Prevention of Stroke*. Springer-Verlag, New York, 1991, pp 83-102.

66. Khaw KT, Barrett-Connor E. Dietary potassium and stroke-associated mortality. A 12-year prospective population study. *N Engl J Med* 1987; **316**: 235-240.

67. Hart RG, Kanter MC. Hematologic disorders and ischemic stroke - a selective review. *Stroke* 1990; **21**: 1111-1121.

68. Kuwabara Y, Ichiya Y, Otsuka M, Masuda K, Ichimiya A, Fujishima M. Cerebrovascular responsiveness to hypercapnia in Alzheimer's dementia and vascular dementia of the Binswanger type. *Stroke* 1992; **23**: 594-598.

69. Tohgi H, Chiba K, Kimura M. Twenty-four-hour variation of blood pressure in vascular dementia of the Binswanger type. *Stroke* 1991; **22**: 603-608.

70. Thomas DJ. Rheology and strokes. *Curr Opin Neurol Neurosurg* 1992; **5**: 44-48.

71. Ott E. Hyperviscosity syndromes. In: Toole JF (ed) *Handbook of Clinical Neurology, Vol 11* **(55)**: Vascular Diseases, Part III. Elsevier Science Publishers, Amsterdam, 1989, pp 483-492.

72. Blondal H, Guomundsson G, Benedikz E, Johannesson G. Dementia in hereditary cystatin C amyloidosis. *Prog Clin Bio Res* 1989; **317**: 157-164.

73. Haan J, Lanser JBK, Zijderveld I, van der Does IGF, Roos RAC. Dementia in hereditary cerebral hemorrhage with amyloidosis - Dutch type. *Arch Neurol* 1990; **47**: 965-967.

74. Levy E, Carman MD, Fernandez-Madrid IJ *et al*. Mutation of the Alzheimer's disease amyloid gene in hereditray cerebral hemorrhage, Dutch type. *Science* 1990; **248**: 1124-1126.

75. Tournier-Lasserve E, Joutel A, Melki J *et al*. Cerebral autosomal dominant arteriopathy with subcortical infarcts and leukoencephalopathy maps to chromosome 19q12. *Nat Genet* 1993; **3**: 256-259.

76. Sourander P, Walinder J. Hereditary multi-infarct dementia. Morphological and clinical studies of a new disease. *Acta Neuropathol* 1977; **39**: 247-254.

77. Baudrimont M, Dubas F, Joutel A, Tournier-Lasserve E, Bousser MG. Autosomal dominant leukoencephalopathy and subcortical ischemic stroke. A clinicopathological study. *Stroke* 1993; **24**: 122-125.

78. Brown WD, Frackowiak RSJ. Cerebral blood flow and metabolism studies in multi-infarct dementia. *Alzheimer Dis Assoc Disord* 1991; **5**: 131-143.

79. Hossmann K-A. Viability thresholds and the penumbra of focal ischemia. *Ann Neurol* 1994; **36**: 557-565.

80. Hirono N, Yamadori A, Komiyama M. Dural arteriovenous fistula: a cause of hypoperfusion-induced intellectual impairment. *Eur Neurol* 1993; **33**: 5-8.

81. Easton JD, Sherman DG. Cervical manipulation and stroke. *Stroke* 1977; **8**: 594-597.

82. Brust JCM. Clinical, radiological, and pathological aspects of cerebrovascular disease associated with drug abuse. *Stroke* 1993; **24[suppl I]**: I-129-I-133.

83. Collaborative Group for the Study of Stroke in Young Woman. Oral contraceptives and stroke in young woman - associated risk factors. *JAMA* 1975; **231**: 718-722.

84. Rockwood K, Parhad I, Hachinski V *et al.* Diagnosis of vascular dementia: consortium of canadian centres for clinical cognitive research concensus statement. *Can J Neurol Sci* 1994; **21**: 358-364.

85. Meyer JS, Judd BW, Tawaklna T, Rogers RL, Mortel KF. Improved cognition after control of risk factors for multi-infarct dementia. *JAMA* 1986; **256**: 2203-2209.

86. Meyer JS, Rogers RL, McClintic K, Mortel KF, Lotfi J. Randomized clinical trial of daily aspirin therapy in multi-infarct dementia - a pilot study. *J Am Geriatr Soc* 1989; **37**: 549-555.

7

NEUROENDOCRINE FACTORS

Bruce S. McEwen

*T*his chapter deals with brain and endocrine mechanisms that are relevant to cognitive function and how these mechanisms participate in changes in cognition during aging. Some comments are based upon animal experimentation that we and other laboratories have been doing over the past 20 years. The focus will be data that are relevant to treatments that might prevent cognitive decline. Intervention early enough may actually make a difference, if it is discovered when and how.

Several years ago Purifoy[1] discussed the endocrine system as one of the main contributors to human variability. Since then much of what is discussed with respect to aging has to do with individual differences in brain and body aging, and it is particularly relevant to discuss endocrine factors. It is the life course of environmental, including hormonal, influences on an individual's genome that determines how each person ages and which disorders will express themselves and when. This chapter focuses on the role of gonadal and adrenal steroids and thyroid hormone in brain development and aging.

THE ENDOCRINE-BRAIN DIALOG

One of the great discoveries of this century has been the fact that the brain controls the endocrine system through the anterior pituitary and posterior lobes of the pituitary gland. The anterior pituitary has a vasculature which then transfers chemical messengers from the median eminence to trigger the secretion of a variety of trophic hormones such as ACTH and the gonadotropins, thyrotropic hormone, prolactin and growth hormone. The posterior pituitary receives nerve endings from the hypothalamus and there releases neuropeptides of important hormones such as antidiuretic hormone, or vasopressin and oxytocin, which have their own very important effects.

The relationship of the brain to the endocrine system is very much a two–way street. This is because the final hormones, such as thyroid hormone, the adrenal steroids and the gonadal steroids, feedback on many organs of the body to convey their own chemical messages. The brain and pituitary gland are targets of these circulating hormones and therefore the neuroendocrine system is subject to feedback regulation and at the same time exerts important influences on brain function and behavior. In fact, the first experiment in the field of endocrinology was published in 1849 by a German anatomist called Berthold,[2] and it was a study of the effects of trans-planting the testes of the rooster into a castrated rooster. Berthold observed that not only did the secondary sex characteristics, the comb and the wattle, return to normal after this testicular transplant, but the behavior of the animal, the crowing, the aggression and the sexual behavior, which had disappeared after castration, returned as well. Berthold inferred that there was a testicular product, which we now know as testosterone, that was affecting the brain. Subsequent work in this century, implanting tiny crystals of testosterone into the brain, has actually demonstrated sites in the brain that are sensitive to these circulating hormones.

HORMONES AND BRAIN DEVELOPMENT

One of the ways that the endocrine system plays a role in defining individual differences has to do with the effects of hormones on development. There are three major examples (Fig. 7.1).

1. The most prominent example has to do with the presence or absence of testos-terone, leading to sexual differentiation, not only of the reproductive organs of the body but also of certain structures within the brain, leading to differences in cognitive function and other aspects of behavior and susceptibility to disease, between males and females.[3,4]

2. Effects of thyroid hormone.[5] The normal state is the so-called euthyroid state, but the normal bell curve distribution of hormonal activity in organisms means that there is a range of secretion of thyroid hormone among individuals, which has extremely important developmental effects, especially early in life. The extreme conditions of being either hypo- or hyperthyroid lead to abnormalities in brain development. There are undoubtedly lesser variations, that may not qualify in the pathologic sense, which can also contribute to differences in the brain structure and function.

3. Stress and stressful experiences early in life. Meaney *et al*[6] showed that early handling of newborn rats, which is a mild stimulation, every day for the first 14 days of neonatal life, resulted in a reduction in the rate of aging of their brains. Brain aging in relation to adrenal steroids and stress is discussed futher later.

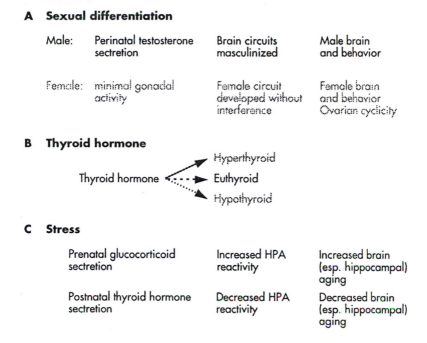

A   Sexual differentiation

Male: Perinatal testosterone   Brain circuits   Male brain
        sectretion   masculinized   and behavior

Female: minimal gonadal   Female circuit   Female brain
         activity   developed without   and behavior
                           interference   Ovarian cyclicity

B   Thyroid hormone

Thyroid hormone → Hyperthyroid / Euthyroid / Hypothyroid

C   Stress

Prenatal glucocorticoid   Increased HPA   Increased brain
sectretion   reactivity   (esp. hippocampal)
                                          aging

Postnatal thyroid hormone   Decreased HPA   Decreased brain
sectretion   reactivity   (esp. hippocampal)
                                            aging

Figure 7.1 – Diagram of the relationships between developmental actions of hormones on brain and their consequences in adult life.
A. Sexual differentiation is the result of actions of testosterone during pre- and postnatal development.
B. Thyroid hormone actions are directed at the 'euthyroid' state, and excess or deficiency of thyroid hormone levels during development has deleterious effects for brain structure and function.
C. Stress acting prenatally, at least in part via glucocorticoid secretion, causes enhanced reactivity of the hypothalamo-pituitary-adrenal (HPA) axis in adult life and leads to faster brain (especially hippocampal) aging. Postnatal 'handling' of rat pups has the opposite effect on HPA reactivity in adult life and can even reverse effects of prenatal stress. Thyroid hormone secretion appears to play a key role in these effects.

HORMONE RECEPTORS AND ACTIONS

Steroid and thyroid hormones bind to receptors inside the cell.[7] Steroid hormones enter cell nuclei and bind to receptor proteins, which then bind directly to regions of the DNA and alter the transcription of genes The brain has receptors for all the major classes of steroid hormones: androgens, estrogens, progestins, glucocorticoids, mineralicorticoids, vitamin D (which is very much a steroid hormone), and thyroid hormone. These are distributed in unique patterns for each of these steroid type, and are expressed and developmentally regulated in individual brain regions, so that the study of this whole system is a very rich and challenging one as it concerns the anatomy of an incredibly complicated structure.

As an example of a hormone effect in the hypothalamus of a female rat, estrogen induces the expression of large numbers of oxytocin receptors in the ventromedial nuclei (VMN).[8] The oxytocin is produced somewhere else in the hypothalamus and the oxytocin nerve endings are actually located in the area adjacent to the VMN. After giving estrogen, oxytocin receptors spread out along the dendrites from the VMN and move toward the area where their synaptic endings which release the oxytocin are present. Blocking oxytocin receptors in the VMN interferes with the expression of sexual behavior in the female rat.

Thus steroid hormones are secreted as part of natural endocrine cycles, and they coordinate the reproductive process with reproductive behavior at different seasons of the year or times of the month.[9] Adrenal steroids are also produced in response to a diurnal clock or rhythm. The level of adrenal steroids, for example, is very important for cognitive alertness at certain times of the day and perhaps somewhat less alertness at others. It is very likely that the deregulation or disruption of adrenal steroid secretion contributes to the cognitive impairments seen in jet-lag.

Hormones, especially the stress hormones, are also secreted as a result of experiences, and stressful experiences in particular. They also play an important role in modulating learning and memory.

FUNCTIONS OF THE HIPPOCAMPUS

Adrenal steroids are implicated in cognitive function, as in the link between the diurnal rhythm and jet-lag. However, in situations of excess adrenal steroid secretion, such as in Cushing's syndrome, in major depressive disorders and with prolonged stressful experiences, cognitive impairment has been demonstrated in experimental animals and in man. With very severe insults, such as stroke or ischemic damage, there are indications that glucocorticoids can exacerbate this effect. Not enough is known about the etiology of degenerative brain disorders such as Alzheimer's disease to understand how stress and adrenal steroids might make a contribution.

The brain structure that really is at center stage for most of the discussion of cognitive function is the hippocampal formation, which gets its name because its shape reminded early neuroanatomists of the seahorse, or hippocampus. The entorhinal cortex is the first input to the hippocampus, which consists of the Ammon's horn and the dentate gyrus. These are distinct parts, the dentate gyrus arising later in development than the Ammon's horn.

The hippocampal formation has many functions in behavior.[10] For example, spatial learning and memory are impaired after hippocampal lesions and so is declarative and episodic memory. Some people talk about working memory as being the flexibility to adapt behavior to a changing situation, and this also is impaired when the hippocampus is damaged. There is something called memory indexing, the idea that the hippocampus, which by no means stores all the memories in the brain, is nevertheless an important way-station in locating where to store a memory and where to retrieve it once it has been stored. The hippocampus is also involved in relating expectancy to reality, in spatial learning and in memory. Finally, the hippocampus plays a very important role in emotional learning and memory in determining the appropriate or inappropriate place to show fear or anxiety.[11,12] If you have been shocked or punished in one environment and you go into that environment again, it is appropriate to be scared; but if you go into a different environment and are still frightened, the response is inappropriate.

THE HIPPOCAMPUS, STRESS AND ADRENAL STEROIDS

In 1968 we discovered that the hippocampal formation of rats and later of rhesus monkeys takes up and concentrates the adrenal steroid, corticosterone, in neurons of the Ammon's horn and the dentate gyrus.[13] The hormone is located in the nuclei of these cells, and all the principal neurons of Ammon's horn and of the dentate gyrus appear to have these steroid receptors.

It took until the late 1970s before some of the functions of these adrenal steroids were realized. These effects are paradoxical, because, on the one hand, adrenal steroids cause damage while, on the other hand, their secretion is essential for survival.[9,14] That is, if you do not have an adrenal cortex, you are very vulnerable to stress. In fact, glucocorticoids have the very important function of containing primary responses within the brain to the activation of various neurotransmitter systems. The analogy is an inflammatory response, where cortisone acts to reduce the inflammation. The inflammatory response is a primary response of the body to an insult or irritation, and glucocorticoids contain this response. They do so in the brain as well, containing not only inflammatory processes by damping activity of a number of neurotransmitter systems.

So the paradox is that adrenal steroids have both protective and damaging actions and the difference between them is one of timing and also duration of exposure. Damage occurs with high levels of adrenal steroids and over long periods of time. Glucocorticoids and mineralocorticoids also play an important role in modulating long-term potentiation which many believe is related to learning and memory. This may have implications for diurnal rhythm and jet-lag because the effects of adrenal steroids are bi-phasic, i.e. low levels facilitate and high levels inhibit.[9,14] Another basic role of physiological levels of adrenal steroids involves the regulation of cell birth and cell death in the dentate gyrus. There is an ongoing turnover of nerve cells in this part of the hippocampal formation which is contained or negatively regulated by circulating adrenal steroids and also by excitatory amino acid neurotransmitters. How this fits into the whole spectrum of the physiology of adrenal steroids is not known but it may be that the process allows the hippocampus to get larger at certain seasons of the year and smaller at others.

The work of Philip Landfield and collaborators showed that in aging 24 month old Fischer rats there is a noticeable reduction in the density of pyramidal neurons in the hippocampal formation.[15,16] Landfield's group did an experiment in which they adrenalectomized rats at mid-life and kept them alive for 6 months, which is no easy feat; they found that the adrenalectomy reduced the rate at which pyramidal neurons were lost. Subsequently, Robert Sapolsky, as a graduate student in our lab at Rockefeller, gave glucocorticoids to young rats for 12 weeks and was able to reproduce this kind of cell loss in young animals, thus inducing a type of premature aging.[1]

Sapolsky went on to study the effects of social stress in vervet monkeys living in social groupings where the subordinate animals received immense amounts of abuse over long periods of time from the dominant animals. He and Hideo Uno, a neuropathologist at the University of Wisconsin, found that pyramidal neurons in a region of the hippocampus, called the CA3, are noticeably absent compared to the non-stressed controls. Thus very severe and prolonged stress may be a factor causing brain damage.[18]

Are these findings of relevance to humans? The answer is not yet known but recent data indicate that 'hippocampal lucency', an indirect measurement of hippocampal volume from measuring ventricular volume next to the hippocampus, is increased in elderly individuals who have some cognitive impairment.[19,20] Following such individuals over a number of years, it has been shown that there is a very high probability that they will go on to develop frank Alzheimer's disease.[21] There is also an increase in hippocampal lucency with age, within decades from the 50s to the 80s and 90's. Normal individuals do eventually show hippocampal atrophy, whereas demented individuals show it much earlier.

Although there is no linkage thus far between hippocampal size, stress or glucocorticoids, there are some strong hints in this direction.

1. Hippocampal lesion size correlates with higher cortisol level in a glucose tolerance test.[22] This links the detection of glucose with the secretion of glucocorticoids and with the volume of the hippocampus and it is an observation that needs to be followed up because there are indications that giving glucose can improve memory.[23,24] The hippocampus, according to Sapolsky's work, is particularly vulnerable to damage resulting from an 'energy crisis', i.e. inadequate glucose stores during heavy activity.[17]

2. In Cushing's disease, it has been found that individuals with a smaller hippocampal volume, as measured by MRI, did worse on verbal recall testing.[25] Also, those who had a smaller hippocampus tended to have higher levels of cortisol in the blood.

3. There are indications that rats stressed for 3 weeks by a restraint stress show atrophy of neurons in the hippocampus and display a reduction in the number of correct choices they make in initially learning a radial arm maze.[14] Also, in eight trials these rats made mistakes earlier when solving this spatial orientation problem. The effects of stress are similar in direction to the effects seen with aging, but they are not as severe.

4. In subordinate tree shrews, a primitive relative of primates, exposed to a dominant animal 1 hour per day over 28 days, there is atrophy of the apical dendrites of pyramidal neurons in the area called the CA3 (Margarinos, McEwan, Flugge and Fuchs, unpublished). As in the rat, the basal dendrites do not show the change after repeated restraint stress. Its only the apical dendrites which shrink and retract.

The atrophy of apical dendrites of hippocampal CA3 pyramidal neurons occurs after giving a rat corticosterone for 3 weeks.[14] Sapolsky used the same dose of corticosterone over 12 weeks to cause pyramidal cell loss. After 3 weeks, we saw no cell loss but a marked atrophy of the apical dendritic tree, and no statistically significant reduction in the basal dendritic tree (Fig.7.2). We believe that the apical dendrites of the CA3 region receive a synaptic input from the dentate gyrus, and this synaptic input, the so-called mossy fiber terminals, releases the neurotransmitter glutamate.

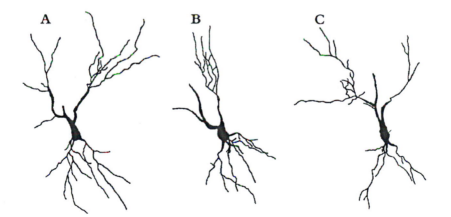

Figure 7.2 – Representative camera lucida drawings of hippocampal CA3 pyramidal neurons from rats undergoing
A. No stress exposure;
B. 21 days of daily restraint stress;
C. Daily stress preceded by Dilantin treatment. Note decrease in number of dendritic branch points in B compared to both A and C. Thus Dilantin blocks dendritic atrophy produced by stress as well as that produced by daily corticosterone treatment.[26]

Glutamate is involved in all of the damaging effects of ischemia, head trauma and seizures but is also a vital neurotransmitter that mediates for example learning, memory and long-term potentiation. As only the apical dendrites atrophy under stress we have conducted a number of experiments to implicate glutamate in the process by which glucocorticoids and stress this atrophy. Dilantin (phenytoin, an antiepileptic drug that blocks the release and certain actions of excitatory amino acids) treatment blocked both the stress effect and the corticosterone effect to cause atrophy of apical dendrites of CA3 pyramidal neurons (Fig. 7.2). Because Dilantin did not block the ability of corticosterone to cause the involution of the thymus, which is another action of glucocorticoids, it is not acting as an anti-glucocorticoid, but rather with regard to glutamate. We then found that NMDA receptors are involved, since an antagonist for this receptor blocked stress-induced atrophy of dendrites.

If glutamate is so important, then where do glucocorticoids act? There are multiple sites where glucocorticoids appear to exert effects on both sides of the glutamatergic synapses.[14] In one study, restraint stress caused a release of glutamate, measured by microdialysis, but adrenalectomized rats did not show stress-induced glutamate release. So regulating the production or release of glutamate is one of the ways glucocorticoid action causes dendritic atrophy, but it is not the only one. Weiland and Orchinik have shown that glucocorticoid treatment decreases the inhibitory tone on neurons in the hippocampus by suppressing GABA receptors and at the same time it elevates expression of the NMDA receptors. It is interesting that glucocorticoids do not reduce the total number of GABA receptors but rather change the subunit composition of the GABA receptors. The GABA receptor is made up of a number of subunits, and they can combine in many different ways to form different kinds of receptors. The resulting receptor, after corticosterone treatment, is less sensitive to benzodiazepines that work synergisitically with GABA to activate this receptor, and is also less sensitive to GABA-active neurosteroids. In other words, GABA receptors in the hippocampus of an animal treated with corticosterone are less sensitive to agents that promote the inhibitory actions of GABA.

Neurosteroids are produced from natural steroids such a progesterone and deoxycorticosterone, and they can be produced in the brain itself.[27] Their structures are such that they do not bind to conventional intracellular receptors but are able to bind to a site on the GABA receptor that synergizes with barbiturates, with benzodiazepines and with the inhibitory transmitter GABA itself, to produce inhibition

In the communication between the dentate gyrus and the CA3 neurons, there is a very important component, an inhibitory interneuron.[14] The mossy fibers not only activate the apical dendrites of the CA3 neurons, but they also activate the interneurons. The interneurons, in turn, produce inhibition at the cell body level. By increasing the NMDA receptor, you would enhance the excitatory and also the atropy-producing effect. If at the same time glucocorticoids are reducing the ability of GABA, the neurosteroids and the benzodiazepines to provide inhibition, a possible source of protection is removed and these cells are left open to overstimulation.

This interaction between excitatory and inhibitory neurons allows for a number of means of intevention to prevent atrophy.[14] Pharmacologic blockade of dendritic atrophy can be accomplished by blocking adrenal steroid synthesis. It can also be accomplished with Dilantin, an NMDA receptor blocker or a benzodiazepine which will enhance the inhibitory system. Therefore if a human brain is undergoing neuronal atrophy, and possibly Cushing's syndrome is an example, there are different strategies for interfering with the degenerative change. It also needs to be mentioned that the atrophy described above, resulting from up to 3 weeks of stress or corticosterone treatment, is a reversible process. It becomes irreversible with the prolongation of these treatments. If this type of atrophy is a forerunner of actual permanent cell loss, we might be able to intervene early enough with some of these pharmacologic treatments.

ESTROGENS AND NON-REPRODUCTIVE BRAIN FUNCTION

Sex hormones are important at every stage of brain development and function: embryonic and neonatal life, during puberty, and in adult life. Both androgens and estrogens act in various sex specific ways. What needs to be appreciated is that the gonadal hormones are important for far more than just reproductive events and reproductive behavior, and their decline later in life or because of ovariectomy can have significant effects on brain structure and function that are only beginning to be realized.

Examples of what estrogens do outside of the area of reproduction include influence on motor activity and improvement of fine motor skills.[28] They also have effects, often inhibitory, on the dopaminergic system and they exacerbate the symptoms of Parkinson's disease, although low doses of estrogen can actually have the opposite effect.

A type of epilepsy, catamenial epilepsy, occurs in some individuals according to the stage of the menstrual cycle.[28] The cause of premenstrual syndrome is not known, but interrupting ovarian cyclicity disrupts the periodic dysphoria. There is more depressive illness in women than in men, and high, pharmacologic doses of estrogen treatment have been shown to reduce depressive symptoms. Recent studies in mice indicate that males and females use functionally distinct pain pathways, and that gonadal steroids, particularly estrogens, play a major role in regulating these pathways.

There are reports of beneficial effects of estrogens, especially in surgical menopause and sometimes in natural menopause, on cognitive performance. There are sex differences in humans and in animals for the strategies used in solving spatial navigation problems. The hippocampus, which is the brain structure central to cognition, shows sex differences in its structure and chemistry. There are indications that estrogens have beneficial effects in dementia.

Besides its very specific effects in the hypothalamus and in preoptic area and amygdala, which are related to reproduction, estrogens effect many of the major, widely-projecting neuronal systems of the brain, such as the noradrenergic, serotinergic, cholinergic and dopaminergic systems. As an example of this, it was found that giving estrogens to an adult female rat induces enzymes for producing acetylcholine, and that these enzymes are induced in the cell body region of the basal forebrain and transported to nerve endings in the cortex and the hippocampus.[2]

Estrogens and the hippocampus

In 1968, Terasawa and Timiras showed that in a female rat, on the day of pro−estrus, when the animal shows ovulation and sex behavior, it is much easier to elicit a seizure by stimulating the dorsal hippocampus. This sensitivity almost immediately disappears and the threshold does not rise again until the next time of ovulation.

Woolley found in looking at the hippocampus that estrogens induce spines, which are tiny structures that receive specialized synaptic inputs that are excitatory and that release glutamate and probably contact NMDA receptors (Fig. 7.3). Estrogen

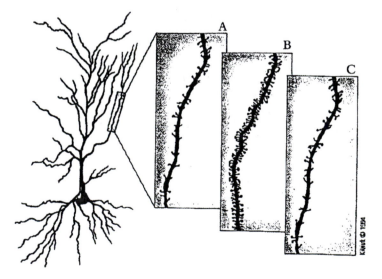

Figure 7.3 − The cyclic variation of dendritic spine density during the estrous cycle on CA1 pyramidal neurons.
A. Diestrus;
B. Proestrus (day of ovulation and sexual activity);
C. Estrus (day of resetting of cycle).[32]

treatment induces a very substantial increase in the density of these spines and of synapses on the spines.[29] She used electron microscopy to show that estrogen treatment increases actual synapse counts on these dendritic spines but does not change the number of synapses on the dendritic shafts. Most of the input to these neurons is glutamatergic, and most of this is on the dendritic spines. There is also noradrenergic, serotonergic and cholinergic input, but it does not seem to be relevant to the induction of new synapses. When Woolley blocked NMDA receptors in female rats receiving estrogen, she prevented the formation of these synapses. This is another example of a collaboration between a steroid hormone and the release of an excitatory amino acid transmitter.[30]

How do these new synapses disappear? Woolley found that spine density rose and fell during the estrous cycle of the female rat, being low on di-estrus, reaching a peak on pro-estrus when the increased seizure susceptibility occurred, and within 12 to 24 hours it disappeared (Fig. 7.3). On the afternoon of pro-estrus, in conjunction with the proestrus LH surge that causes ovulation and the appearance of sexual receptivity in a female rat, there is a massive surge of progesterone. Woolley was able to show that synapse disappearance could be blocked with RU486, an antagonist of the intracellular progesterone receptor that is very effective in terminating a pregnancy.[31]

This means that there must be an estrogen inducible progestin receptor as well as an estrogen receptor somewhere in the hippocampus. The CA1 pyramidal neurons, where the new synapses are formed with the aid of the NMDA receptor and estradiol, do not contain any estrogen or progestin receptors at all. The only estrogen receptors we can detect in the adult hippocampus are present in GABA containing interneurons. Thus our conclusion is that estrogen and progesterone, acting on these inhibitory neurons, can regulate the formation and destruction of synapses transynaptically in pyramidal neurons.[29] One way this could happen is by synapsing on another GABA interneuron which does not have these estrogen receptors and by inhibiting this inhibitory interneuron you disinhibit and tend to facilitate or excite the pyramidal cells.

What do these actions of estrogens have to do with human aging? There is an increasing incidence of dementia with age and women have a higher incidence than men, especially in the age range 65-74.[33] In women the menopause is accompanied by a profound reduction in ovarian steroid secretion and in males there is a reduction in testosterone levels with age. The lack of or reduction in gonadal hormones certainly might make some contribution to increased dementia.

Fillit conducted the first study of estrogen therapy in a group of women with late onset Alzheimer's-type dementia. He found that in 4 of 7 patients treated with an oral estrogen therapy, there was a significant elevation of the Mini Mental Status score and this even outlasted the decline in estrogens at the termination of the trial.[34] This finding was replicated by a Japanese group, suggesting that at least from a pharmacologic standpoint, estrogen therapy is worth considering.[35] Recently a Henderson and Paganini-Hill, measured Mini Mental Status Examination scores in women with an Alzheimer's-type dementia and showed that those on estrogen replacement therapy had a higher score than those who were not.[36] Paginini-Hill and Henderson also demonstrated in a retrospective death certificate study that the incidence of Alzheimer's-type dementia as a cause of death in women receiving estrogen replacement therapy for varying periods of time before their death, was much reduced in women receiving ERT relatively longer.[37] However, another study from Seattle, reported no such effect.[38] In this study it is interesting to note that there was a much higher incidence of estrogen replacement therapy in both the control and demented groups. There was also an education effect which was not evident in the Paganini-Hill and Henderson study. Finally, there was also a higher incidence of surgical menopause in the Alzheimer's group then in the control group. Many issues that remain to be resolved in these kinds of epidemiological studies.

CONCLUSION

Studies on experimental animals, which began as an exercise in basic research on how hormones affect the brain, are now showing some clues about mechanisms relating to human aging and possible causes of brain damage and dementia. This chapter has focused on the hippocampus, a brain region that is very important for various aspects of memory. It is also a brain region that is extremely vulnerable to many insults, such as head trauma, stroke, epilepsy and chronic stress as well as changes during aging.

The hippocampus responds to adrenal steroids that are secreted during the diurnal rhythm and stress, and these hormones modulate neuron structure and excitability, but they also participate in stress-induced atrophy of neuronal processes along with endogenous excitatory neurotransmitters. Strategies to reduce hippocampal atrophy may be useful as a means of improving cognitive function in the elderly and as a way of preventing more permanent changes such as neuronal loss. The loss of gonadal steroids or their severe reduction in the female menopause, and also in males as they age, may have some adverse effects on brain function. Studies in animals indicate that maintenance of normal connectivity through synapses in the hippocampus is an important action of estrogen, and also that the cholinergic systems as well as noradrenergic, serotonergic and dopaminergic systems, are also affected by ovarian steroids. The male brain appears to respond in somewhat different ways to these hormones, although it does respond to estrogens as well as androgens. So perhaps one should think about androgen replacement therapy for males and estrogen therapy for females. Forthcoming large-scale clinical trials will inform us whether estrogen therapy for women is warranted in cases of memory impairment and as a prophylactic for dementia.

REFERENCES

1. Purifoy F. Endocrine-environment interaction in human variability. *Ann Rev Anthropol* 1981; **10:** 141–162.

2. Berthold AA.Transplantation der Hoden. *Arch Anat Physiol Wiss Med* 1849; **16:** 42–60.

3. Goy R, McEwen BS. *Sexual Differentiation of the Brain*. MIT Press, Cambridge, 1980.

4. Kimura D. Sex differences in the brain. *Sci Am* 1992; **267:** 119–125.

5. Gould E, Woolley C, McEwen BS. The hippocampal formation: morphological changes induced by thyroid, gonadal and adrenal hormones. *Psychoneuroendocrinology* 1991; **16:** 67–84.

6   Meaney M, Aitken D, Berkel H, Bhatnager S, Sapolsky R. Effect of neonatal handling of age-related impairments associated with the hippocampus. *Science* 1988; **239:** 766–768.

7. Yamamoto K. Steroid receptor regulated transcription of specific genes and gene networks. *Ann Rev Genet* 1985; **19:** 209–252.

8. Schumacher M, Coirini H, Flanagan L, Frankfurt M, Pfaff D, McEwen BS. Ovarian steroid modulation of oxytocin receptor binding in the ventromedial hypothalamus. In: Pedersen C, Caldwell J, Jirikowski G, Insel T (eds), *Oxytocin in Maternal, Sexual and Social Behaviors. Ann NY Acad Sci*, New York, 1992, pp 374–386.

9. McEwen BS, Sakai RR, Spencer RL. Adrenal steroid effects on the brain: versatile hormones with good and bad effects. In: Schulkin J (ed) *Hormonally-Induced Changes in Mind and Brain*. Academic Press, San Diego, 1993, pp 157–189.

10. Eichenbaum H, Otto T, Cohen NJ. Two functional components of the hippocampal memory system. *Behav Brain Sci* 1994; **17:** 449–518.

11. Phillips RG, LeDoux JE. Differential contribution of amygdala and hippocampus to cued and contextual fear conditioning. *Behav Neurosci* 1992; **106:** 274–285.

12. LeDoux JE. In search of an emotional system in the brain: leaping from fear to emotion and consciousness. In: Gazzaniga M (ed) *The Cognitive Neurosciences*. MIT Press, Cambridge, 1995, pp 1049–1061.

13. McEwen BS, DeKloet ER, Rostene W. Adrenal steroid receptors and actions in the nervous system. *Physiol Rev* 1968; **66:** 1121–1188.

14. McEwen BS, Albeck D, Cameron H et al. Stress and the brain: A paradoxical role for adrenal steroids. In: Litwack GD (ed) *Vitamins and Hormones*. Academic Press, San Diego, 1995, pp 371–402.

15. Landfield P. Modulation of brain aging correlates by long-term alterations of adrenal steroids and neurally-active peptides. *Prog Brain Res* 1987; **72:** 279–300.

16. Landfield PW, Eldridge JC. Evolving aspects of the glucocorticoid hypothesis of brain aging: Hormonal modulation of neuronal calcium homeostasis. *Neurobiol Aging* 1994; **15:** 579–588.

17. Sapolsky R. *Stress, the Aging Brain and the Mechanisms of Neuron Death*. MIT Press, Cambridge, 1992, pp 1–423.

18. Uno H, Ross T, Else J, Suleman M, Sapolsky R. Hippocampal damage associated with prolonged and fatal stress in primates. *J Neurosci* 1989; **9:** 1705–1711.

19. Convit A, de Leon MJ, Tarshish C et al. Hippocampal volume losses in minimally impaired elderly. *Lancet* 1995; **345:** 266

20. Golomb J, Kluger A, de Leon MJ et al. Hippocampal formation size in normal humag aging: a correlate of delayed secondary memory performance. *Learning Memory* 1994; **1:** 45–54.

21. De Leon MJ, Golomb J, George AE *et al*. The radiologic prediction of Alzheimer disease: the atrophic hippocampal formation. *Am J Neuroradiol* 1993; **14**: 897–906.

22. DeLeon MJ, McRae T, Tsai JR *et al*. Abnormal cortisol response in alzheimer's disease linked to hippocampal atrophy. *Lancet* 1988; 391–392.

23. Kopf SR, Baratti CM. Memory-improving actions of glucose: Involvement of a central cholinergic muscarinic mechanism. *Behav Neural Biol* 1992; **62**: 237–243.

24. Craft S, Newcomer J, Kanne S *et al*. Memory improvement following induced hyperinsuline-mia in Alzheimer's disease. *Neurobiol Aging* 1995; **17**: 123–130.

25. Starkman M, Gebarski S, Berent S, Schteingart D. Hippocampal formation volume, memory dysfunction, and cortisol levels in patients with Cushing's syndrome. *Biol Psychiat* 1992; **32**: 756–765.

26. Watanabe Y, Gould E, Cameron HA, Daniels DC, McEwen BS. Phenytoin prevents stress- and corticosterone-induced atrophy of CA3 pyramidal neurons. *Hippocampus* 1992; **2**: 431–436.

27. Baulieu EE, Robel P. Neurosteroids: A new brain function? *J Steroid Biochem Mol Biol* 1990; **37**: 395–403.

28. McEwen BS. Ovarian steroids have diverse effects on brain structure and function. In: Berg G Hammat M (Eds) *The Modern Management of the Menopause*, 1994, pp 269–278. Parthenon NY.

29. McEwen BS, Gould E, Orchinik M, Weiland NG, Woolley CS. Oestrogens and the structural and functional plasticity of neurons: implications for memory, ageing and neurodegenerative processes. In: Goode J (ed) *Ciba Foundation Symposium #191 The Non-reproductive Actions of Sex Steroids*. CIBA Foundation, London, 1995.

30. Woolley C, McEwen BS. Estradiol regulates hippocampal dendritic spine density via an N-methyl-D-aspartate receptor dependent mechanism. *J Neurosci* 1994; **14**: 7680–7687.

31. Woolley C, McEwen BS. Roles of estradiol and progesterone in regulation of hippocampal dendritic spine density during the estrous cycle in the rat. *J Comp Neurol* 1993; **336**: 293–306.

32. McEwen BS, Schmeck HM. *The Hostage Brain*. *Rockefeller* University Press, New York,1995.

33. Birge SJ. The role of estrogen deficiency in the aging central nervous system. In: Lobo RA (ed) *Treatment of the Postmenopausal Woman: Basic and Clinical Aspects*. Raven Press Inc, New York, 1994, pp 153–157.

34. Fillit H, Weinreb H, Cholst I, Luine V, McEwen BS, X, Zabriskie J. Observations in a preliminary open trial of estradiol therapy for senile dementia - Alzheimer's type. *Psychoneuroendocrinology* 1986; **11**: 337–345.

35. Honjo H, Ogino Y, Naitoh K Okada H. In vivo effects by estrone sulfate on the central nervous system-senile dementia. *J Steroid Biochem* 1989; **34**: 521–525.

36. Henderson VW, Paganini-Hill A, Emanuel CK, Dunn ME, Buckwalter JG. Estrogen replacement therapy in older women: Comparisons between Alzheimer's disease cases and non demented control subjects. *Arch Neurol* 1994; **51**: 896–900.

37. Paganini-Hill A, Henderson VW. Estrogen deficiency and risk of Alzheimer's disease in women. *Am J Epidemiol* 1994; **3**: 3–16.

38. Brenner DE, Kukull WA, Stergachis A et al. Postmenopausal estrogen replacement therapy and the risk of alzheimer's disease: A population-based case-control study. *Am J Epidemiol* 1994; **140**: 262–267.

8

DELIRIUM AND COGNITIVE DECLINE

Does delerium lead to dementia ?

Sharon K Inouye

D elirium, described as an acute disorder of attention and global cognitive functioning, has assumed particular importance in industrialized societies, with their increasing proportion of elderly citizens. The old–old group (> 75 years old) is the most rapidly growing sector of the United States population, and is particularly vulnerable to developing delirium during acute illness and hospitalization. Previous studies have estimated occurrence rates for delirium from 14 to 56% of elderly hospitalized patient's,[1-18] with associated mortality rates from 10 to 65%. [1,3,4,15,19-28] Delirium is also associated with increased rates of morbidity, functional decline, nursing home placement, and with longer, costlier hospitalizations.[19-33] Levkoff et al[1] have estimated that if the length of stay of each delirious hospitalized elderly patient could be reduced by just one day, the savings to Medicare would amount to $1 to $2 billion (1986 US dollars) per year. This extrapolation highlights the vast economic and health policy implications of delirium.

The problem of delirium in hospitalized elderly patients has assumed particular importance since patients aged 65 years and older account for more than 40% of all inpatient days of hospital care.[34] Based on US vital health statistics,[35] 35.4% of the US population aged 65 years and older was hospitalized during 1993. Using current estimates of 20% of all hospitalized elderly patients presenting with or developing delirium during hospitalization,[1-18] the annual occurrence rates of delirium extrapolated to the larger population of all US elderly persons is 7%, or 70 cases per 1000 persons each year. With these extrapolations, delirium complicates hospital stays for at least 2.2 million persons, involving over 17.5 million inpatient days.

Delirium is clearly an important contributor to acute cognitive decline, and warrants attention as a substantial public health problem in its own right. Moreover, delirium may lead to cognitive impairment and to dementia. This as yet controversial area of the relationship of delirium to chronic cognitive impairment will be the focus of this chapter. The goals of this chapter are to synthesize the existing medical literature in this area, particularly to address:

1. The evidence on the inter-relationship of delirium and dementia;

2. The evidence on whether delirium itself leads to chronic, irreversible cognitive impairment.

PATHOPHYSIOLOGY OF DELIRIUM

The pathophysiology of delirium remains poorly understood. Most investigators hypothesize that delirium is a functional rather than structural lesion.[36] Electroencephalographic studies document the global functional derangements that occur with delirium, characterized by generalized slowing of cortical background (alpha) activity.[37] The leading current hypothesis views delirium as the final common pathway of many different pathogenic mechanisms, as outlined in Table 8.1. Each case of delirium is likely to involve one or more of these mechanisms. Lipowski[55] and Francis[36] have summarized the leading hypothesis on pathophysiology of delirium, and postulate that delirium is most likely the result of widespread reduction in cerebral oxidative metabolism with resultant failure of cholinergic transmission.

Of particular importance here is the fact that several of these basic mechanisms may not be completely reversible, such as those resulting in hypoxemic damage. In addition, the 'dose' and duration of the noxious insult(s) may also exert great influence on the reversibility of the delirium.

Ultimately, however, the basic pathophysiology of delirium remains unclear and poorly investigated. Methodologically rigorous studies (e.g. positron emission tomography, single photon emission computed tomography, neurotransmitter, neurophysiologic) to clarify the underlying pathogenetic mechanisms of delirium are greatly needed.

ETIOLOGY OF DELIRIUM

Delirium defies the classic disease model and the tendency to look for single causes of disease. In fact, delirium is rarely caused by a single factor, but rather represents an intrinsically multifactorial syndrome.[56] The development of delirium involves a complex inter-relationship between a vulnerable host and precipitating factors, or noxious insults. Patients who are highly vulnerable to delirium (e.g. cognitively impaired, severely ill) may be thrown into delirium with precipitating factors even of mild degree. Conversely, patients with low vulnerability would be very resistant to the development of delirium, even with noxious insults.

Table 8.1 – Pathophysiology of delirium*

Hypothesis	Evidence
Reduction of cerebral oxidative metabolism	• The clinical and EEG manifestations of delirium were reversed with experimental interventions including oxygen for hypoxemia, glucose for hypoglycemia, and transfusions for anemia.[37,38]
Reduction of cholinergic transmission,	• Drug-induced anticholinergic intoxication (clinical and experimental) results in the attentional, cognitive and EEG manifestations of delirium, which can be reversed by cholinesterase inhibitors such as physostigmine.[39,40]
	• Acetylcholine synthesis decreases with hypoxia and hypoglycemia. The relative deficiency in the brain of acetylcholine appears to be a common denominator in many toxic-metabolic encephalopathies.[41,42]
	• Serum anticholinergic activity correlates with delirium in hospitalized medical patients[43], post-operative[44] and post-electroconvulsive therapy[45] patients.
Other mediators: Cerebrospinal fluid (CSF) • beta-endorphin • somatostatin	• Koponen *et al*[46,47] found decreased CSF levels of beta-endorphin and somatostatin in delirious patients compared with age-matched controls, which failed to normalize after 2 weeks and declined further at 1 year. Review of the data suggests underlying dementia (which predisposed to delirium) was the major factor determining these levels.
Humoral • lymphokines	• In animal studies,[48] intraventricular injection of interleukin-1 results in clinical and EEG manifestations of delirium. In patients receiving chemotherapy with alpha interferon, interleukin-2 and lymphokine-activated killer cells,[49-51] delirium is a common complication which is dose-related and resolves once treatment is stopped. Thus, lymphokines may play an important role in delirium associated with infectious and inflammatory diseases.
• other (tryptophan, cortisol, beta-endorphin, phenylalanine metabolites)[52-54]	• Individual studies have been limited by small sample sizes, lack of follow-up, and inadequate control for confounding effects of severe illness and underlying dementia.

* Summarized from Francis[36], Lipowski[55], and original articles cited.

The conditions associated with delirium cover a broad range of medical conditions (Table 8.2). It is important to note that not all of these conditions are reversible (such as structural neurologic lesions); in addition, it may not always be possible to alter the patient's vulnerability or to remove all noxious insults. Thus, depending on the underlying etiologies, all cases of delirium may not be reversible

INTER-RELATIONSHIP OF DELIRIUM AND DEMENTIA

The strong inter-relationship of delirium and dementia is amply supported by the medical literature and clinical experience. First, dementia is well-recognized to be an important risk factor for delirium, and provides the substrate for delirium in up to two-thirds of cases.[1,36,56] The literature strongly supports the predisposing role of

Table 8.2 – Etiological factors for delirium

Drugs/Intoxication/Withdrawal

- Sedative-hypnotics; narcotics; anticholinergics; cimetidine; steroids
- Alcohol
- Withdrawal syndromes

Infections

- Systemic: pneumonia, urinary tract infection, sepsis
- Intracranial: encephalitis, meningitis

Metabolic Disorders

- Electrolyte imbalance (sodium, calcium)
- Acid-base disorder
- Volume depletion
- Hypo- and hyperglycemia
- Endocrinopathies (thyroid, parathyroid, adrenal)
- Vitamin deficiencies (thiamine, B12)
- Hypo- and hyperthermia

Systemic Illnesses

- Cardiovascular: myocardial infarction, cognitive heart failure, arrhythmia
- Respiratory failure
- Uremia
- Hepatic encephalopathy

Neurologic Diseases

- Cerebrovascular disorders: thrombosis, embolism, vasculitis, aneurysm
- Space-occupying lesions: neoplasm, subdural hematoma
- Epilepsy (ictal and post-ictal state)

dementia and other structural brain abnormalities in the development of delirium in elderly patients,[55,57,58] perhaps due to a loss of physiological reserve capacity in the face of acute insults - such as medical illness or psychoactive medications.

Although delirium and dementia have been defined as separate conditions in the medical and psychiatric literature, several points of evidence suggest an overlap of these two conditions.[56] Are they two separate conditions, or do they represent two ends of a continuum of cognitive impairment? 'Reversible dementia'[59-63] and 'subacute delirium' are clinical entities that blur the distinctions between these two conditions. Although chronic and irreversible in the vast majority, approximately 5-10% of dementia cases will have a reversible etiology. Subacute delirium, with continuing symptoms over months, has been increasingly recognized in recent studies[64,65] - suggesting that delirium may be far more persistent that previously believed. Thus, there is no question that delirium and dementia are highly inter-related.

Hypotheses for relationship

The question is: does delirium itself lead to chronic cognitive impairment and, ultimately, dementia? The long-standing dogma has been that delirium is reversible, and that all of its symptoms and manifestations should reverse within a relatively short period of time (i.e. days to weeks). However, the evidence of the inter-relationship of delirium and dementia has led investigators to hypothesize several ways delirium may be related to dementia:

1. *Delirium may simply represent worsening dementia.*

   The worsening may be temporary, or may herald a more rapid future decline.

2. *Delirium may unmask an unrecognized dementia.*

   Delirium, which often occurs in the face of acute medical illness, may serve as a vehicle for detection - bringing the patient to medical attention or closer observation during hospitalization. Under this hypothesis, delirium and dementia remain distinct entities, but delirium serves to bring dementia to clinical recognition.

3. *Delirium itself leads to chronic cognitive impairment.*

   Delirium results in irreversible neurologic impairment and structural damage.

A detailed review of the current evidence is needed to evaluate these hypotheses.

Evidence for a relationship

Duration and persistence of delirium

Recent studies on the duration and persistence of delirium symptoms (Table 8.3), document that delirium may be much more persistent than was previously believed.

Table 8.3 – Studies on duration and persistence of delerium

Reference	Population	Method for detection of delirium	Results	Comments
Rockwood 1993[65]	Acute-care Geriatric Assessment Unit, N = 173 (48 (28%) with delirium during hospitalization).	Delirium Symptom Rating Scale[85]	Mean duration of delirium 8 ± 9 days. Complete symptom resolution by discharge in 19/48 (40%).	Measurements and criteria to establish baseline cognitive function and dementia not specified.
Levkoff 199264	Hospitalized medical and surgical patients (65 years, N = 325 (125(38%) with delirium during hospitalization)	Delirium Symptom Interview[78]	Complete symptom resolution by discharge in 5/125 (4%); by 3 mos. in 20.8% and by 6 mos. in 17.7%. No longer met DSM-III criteria for delirium by discharge in 38/125 (30%); by 3 mos. in 63% and by 6 mos. in 69%.	Preexisting cognitive impairment relied on chart review only. No standardized method to detect preexisting cognitive impairment or dementia.
Koponen 1989[66]	Psychogeriatric unit, patients (60 years, N = 70 delirious patients	DSM-III criteria for delirium	Mean duration of delirium 20 days, range 3–81 days.	Detailed assessments carried out to establish baseline cognitive status.
Koizumi 1988 [67]	Hospitalized patients receiving psychiatric consultation, ages 18–89 years, N = 66 delirious patients	DSM-III criteria for delirium	Mean duration of 25.7 (4.6 (SE) days in 35 patients with uncorrected electrolyte disorders, as compared with mean of 9.4 (1.9 (SE) days in 18 patients with corrected electrolyte disorders. Mean duration of 25.0 (6.6 (SE) days in 13 cases without electrolyte imbalance.	Methods to determine baseline cognitive function, and to determine resolution of delirium symptoms not specified.
Sirois 1988[68]	Hospitalized patients referred to consult liaison psychiatry service, N=100 delirious patients	DSM-III criteria for delirium	Duration of delirium was (4 days in 65%, 5–10 days in 20%, and 10–30 days in 15%.	Retrospective chart review only. Methods to determine baseline cognitive function and to determine resolution of delirium symptoms not specified.

In fact, durations of 30 days or more are not unusual according to these studies. Although some of these studies contain methodologic limitations, such as lack of specification of the methods to establish baseline cognitive status and resolution of delirium symptoms, they lend strong support for the potentially long persistence of delirium at least in some cases.

Furthermore, these recent studies support observations by Lipowski[55] that delirium may be followed by a prolonged transitional phase (which includes abnormalities of cognition, affect, or behavior) before full recovery. Thus, persistent and partial (incomplete) manifestations of delirium may be quite common - as supported by the work of Levkoff et al.[64]

Outcomes of delirium

A review of studies of delirium outcomes since 1970 is presented in Table 8.4. In nearly all of these studies, delirium is associated with poor outcomes (i.e. increased mortality, prolonged length of hospital stay, increased rates of institutional placement, functional and cognitive decline) - both at hospital discharge and longer-term follow-up (1 month to 2 years). Clearly, delirium is associated with a poor prognosis. However, it remains unclear whether the delirium itself determines the poor prognosis or whether delirium simply serves as a marker identifying a patient with poor prognostic features due to severe illness, comorbidity, dementia, functional impairment, advanced age, and the like. Unfortunately, many of these studies failed to adequately control for these potential confounders in their analyses and therefore, the independent contribution of delirium to these poor outcomes cannot be determined. Even in studies that did control for these factors, the results remain unclear, since many outcomes (such as mortality) were relatively infrequent, resulting in an increased opportunity for a beta-error.

Overall, taken as a group, however, these studies provide substantial evidence that delirium does contribute to long-term detrimental outcomes, and that these detrimental effects may persist far beyond the identified acute episode. In addition, these studies strongly suggest that delirium has greater detrimental effects in patients with underlying degrees of cognitive impairment.

Re-examining the hypotheses

1. Delirium may simply represent worsening dementia.

This hypothesis represents a dangerous oversimplification, which should be dispelled. Delirium and dementia are considered and should remain clinically distinct syndromes, each with its unique clinical characteristics, pathophysiology, management, and prognosis. Most importantly, delirium should be treated as a potential medical emergency, which warrants immediate attention to prevent the associated high rates of morbidity and mortality.

Table 8.4 – Studies on outcome of delirium

Reference	Population	Method for detection of delirium	Delirium outcomes	Comments
Marcantonio 1994[69]	Elective noncardiac surgical patients > 50 years, N = 1341 (117 (9%) developed postoperative delirium)	Confusion Assessment Method[77]	• **Hospital outcomes:** Patients with delirium had significantly higher rates of death (4% vs. 0.2%), discharge to long-term care or rehabilitative facility (36% vs. 11%), and longer mean LOS (15 vs. 7 days), compared to patients without delirium.	Analyses for delirium outcomes did not control for potential confounders, e.g, illness severity, comorbidity, baseline cognitive and functional status.
Pompei 1994[70]	Medical and surgical patients from a university teaching hospital ≥ 65 years, N=432 (64 (15%) with delirium during hospitalization)	Confusion Assessment Method[77]	• **Mortality:** Delirium cases had significantly higher rates of mortality in-hospital (11% vs. 2%) and within 3 months after discharge (11% vs. 3%). After adjusting for comorbidity, the former association remained significant; the latter did not. • **LOS:** of delirium cases was significantly prolonged beyond the DRG-associated LOS. • **Functional status:** not significantly changed (baseline to 3 months after discharge) between delirious and non-delirious subjects.	Functional status at discharge not evaluated.
Murray 1993[71]	Medical and surgical patients (65 years, N = 325 (125 (38%) with delirium during hospitalization), 30% admitted from nursing home	Delirium Symptom Interview[78]	• **Functional outcomes:** Strong univariate association between incident delirium and functional decline (admission to 3 months after discharge). Delirium persists as sole predictor of functional decline at 3 months, after controlling for pre-existing cognitive impairment, age, sex, comorbidity.	Functional decline persisted at 6 months after hospital discharge. Large number of nursing home patients in sample.

Table 8.4 – Continued

Reference	Population	Method for detection of delirium	Delirium outcomes	Comments
Levkoff 1992[64]	Same population as Murray 1993[71]	Same as above	• **Mortality:** Delirium cases had higher 6 month mortality (26% vs. 13%). After adjusting for age, sex, preexisting cognitive impairment, and illness severity, delirium failed to retain effect on survival. • **LOS:** Delirium contributed to significantly longer average hospital stays, even after adjusting for age, sex, preexisting cognitive impairment, and illness severity. ∘ **Institutional placement:** Delirium cases (from community sample) were far more likely to be institutionalized (44% vs. 7%). Delirium persists as the sole predictor of institutional placement, even after adjusting for age, sex, preexisting cognitive impairment, and illness severity.	Preexisting cognitive impairment determined by chart review. Presence of dementia may have been underestimated and influenced results attributed to delirium.

Table 8.4 – Continued

Reference	Population	Method for detection of delirium	Delirium outcomes	Comments
Francis 1992[72]	Medical patients (70 years, N = 229 (50 (22%) with delirium during hospitalization)	DSM-III-R criteria for delirium	• **Mortality:** 2-year mortality was 39% for delirium cases *vs.* 23% for controls (p =.03). After controlling for comorbidity, baseline cognitive and functional status, delirium failed to have independent effect on survival • **Loss of independent community living (at 2 years):** delirium remained a strong predictor, after controlling for cancer, age, marital status. • **Cognitive decline:** delirium cases had significantly greater cognitive decline at 2 years, adjusting for age, sex, baseline cognitive status.	Relatively small numbers of delirium cases surviving at 2 years (N = 11).
Williams Russo 1992[73]	Elective bilateral total knee replacement patients (58 years, N = 51 (21(41%) developed postoperative delirium)	DSM-III-R criteria for delirium	• **Hospital outcomes:** all delirium cases resolved within 7 days. No differences in LOS and achievement of physical therapy goals in delirious and non-delirious patients.	High-functioning, independent patients at baseline, with no dementia.
Brannstrom 1991[33]	Hip fracture patients with mean age 78.2 years, N = 35 (15(43%) developed post-operative "delirium")	Organic Brain Syndrome Scale[79]	• **Functional outcomes:** Confused patients were more impaired at baseline than non-confused patients. However, the confused patients declined further by 6 months post-fracture, whereas the non-confused patients improved to their baseline functioning.	Outcome not clearly defined. Confused patients included dementia patients, which may have determined outcomes. Small sample size limitations.

Table 8.4 – Continued

Reference	Population	Method for detection of delirium	Delirium outcomes	Comments
Francis 1990[18]	Same population as above, Francis 1992[72]	Same as above, Francis 1992[72]	**Hospital Outcomes** *LOS:* Delirious patients had significantly longer LOS (12.1 vs. 7.2 days), a difference that persisted even after controlling for illness severity, baseline cognitive and functional status and fever. *Mortality:* Significantly higher mortality in delirious patients (8% vs. 1%); other factors no adjusted for. *Institutional placement:* Significantly higher placement rates in delirious patients (16% vs. 3%); other factors not adjusted for. **Six-month outcomes** *Mortality:* 6-month mortality for delirious patients not significantly higher (14% vs. 10%). Once illness severity controlled for, delirium not a significant predictor of 6-month survival (RR=1.8), 95% CI 0.8–4.2). *Institutional placement:* significantly higher rates in delirious patients (12% vs. 5%); other factors not controlled for. *Functional and cognitive outcomes:* No significant differences in rates of ADL or MMSE decline in delirious vs. non-delirious patients.	Relatively small numbers of patients with death and institutional placement.

Table 8.4 – Continued

Reference	Population	Method for detection of delirium	Delirium outcomes	Comments
Rockwood 1990[32]	Medical patients at 2 teaching hospitals (65 years, N = 80) (13 (16%) with delirium during hospitalization)	DSM-III criteria for delirium	**• LOS:** Patients with delirium had an odds ratio of 18.38 for having a delay in discharge and prolonged LOS.	Independent effect of delirium, controlling for other confounders (age, dementia illness severity) not indicated in these analyses.
Koponen 1989[66]	Psychogeriatric unit, patients (60 years, N = 70 delirious patients	DSM-III criteria for delirium	**• Functional and cognitive outcomes:** MMSE and activities of daily living declined substantially at 1-year follow-up in group with underlying dementia. No decline in MMSE in group without underlying dementia.	Underlying dementia in 57 (81%) patients likely to have influenced outcomes. No control groups for comparison; difficult to determine independent effect of delirium.
Magaziner 1989[31]	Hip fracture patients (65 years, N = 814 (157 (19%) with 'delirium' on admission; including 61 with 'delirium without dementia'	Disorientation on admission	**• Mortality:** Patients with 'delirium' on admission (without dementia) had a relative risk for mortality of 3.2 at 3 months, 3.5 at 6 months, and 3.1 at 12 months after hip fracture, compared with patients who were not disoriented.	Ratings of delirium and dementia based on chart review only. Substantial misclassification likely. Adjusted relative risk for delirium, controlling for age, sex, comorbidity, dementia—not given.

Table 8.4 – Continued

Reference	Population	Method for detection of delirium	Delirium outcomes	Comments
Rogers 1989[74]	Elective joint replacement patients (60 years, N = 46 (13 (26%) developed post-operative delirium)	DSM-III criteria for delirium	• **LOS:** delirious patients stayed 1.4 days longer than non-delirious patients, but difference not statistically significant. • **Functional outcomes:** delirious patients showed no improvement in mean function at 6 months post surgery. In a matched subgroup, control patients without delirium improved in functioning.	High-functioning patients at baseline, with no dementia
Gustafson 1988[75]	Hip fracture patients (65 years, N = 111 (68 (61%) admitted with or developed delirium during hospitalization)	Modified Organic Brain Syndrome Scale[79]	• **LOS:** In non-demented patients (and overall), the mean LOS was significantly longer for delirious patients (21.7 vs. 13.5 days) • **Mortality, postoperative complications, institutional placement, poor rehabilitation result:** were significantly higher in delirious patients	Confounding factors (e.g., illness severity, dementia, baseline ADL, age) not controlled for in analyzing outcomes.

Table 8.4 – Continued

Reference	Population	Method for detection of delirium	Delirium outcomes	Comments
Levkoff 1988[76]	Medical and surgical patients (60 years, N = 1285 (117 (9%) with discharge diagnosis of delirium)	Discharge diagnosis of delirium	• **Hospital outcomes** *Mortality:* delirium cases had significantly higher rates of death (13% *vs.* 5%) *Other:* delirium cases had significantly longer LOS (23.7 *vs.* 13.6 days) and higher costs ($17,377 *vs.* $11,946). No significant differences in rate of ICU admission.	Many cases of delirium are not coded as discharge diagnoses; misclassification bias likely. Analyses did not control for confounding effects of age, illness severity, comorbidity, dementia, ADLs.
Thomas 1988[30]	Medical patients, all ages, N = 133 (20 (15%) with delirium during hospitalization)	DSM-III criteria for delirium	• **Hospital outcomes** *LOS:* Geometric mean LOS significantly longer in delirious patients (11.5 *vs.* 7.4 days). After controlling for DRG-predicted LOS, delirium group had a mean of 13 excess days, compared with 3 excess days in non-delirious group. *Mortality:* Significantly more deaths in delirium group (65% *vs.* 4%).	Baseline cognitive function not indicated. Other than DRG group, analyses did not control for confounding effects of age, illness severity, comorbidity, dementia, ADLs.

Table 8.4 – Continued

Reference	Population	Method for detection of delirium	Delirium outcomes	Comments
Fields 1986[29]	Medical patients, all ages, N = 116 (23 (20%) with cognitive impairment on admission).	"Impaired" patients defined as those with MMSE < 24	• **Hospital outcomes** *Mortality:* "Impaired" patients had significantly higher morbidity (39% *vs.* 18%) and mortality (17% *vs.* 5%) rates than iintactf patients. However, these differences do not persist after controlling for illness severity, medical stability, reason for admission, and comorbidity. *LOS:* "Impaired" patients had significantly longer LOS (35.4 *vs.* 11.8 days), although much of this time spent awaiting placement. *Other:* Significantly more "impaired" patients discharged to nursing home or hospice (26% *vs.* 5%), or home with assistance (32% *vs.* 1%) compared with "intact" patients.	"Impaired" group included both delirious and demented patients. Only in-hospital morbidity and mortality analyses controlled for confounders.
Rabins 1982[24]	Hospitalized patients referred for psychiatric consultation, all ages, with delirium or dementia, N = 73 (48% (66%) with delirium)	Delirium defined as MMSE < 24 and abnormal level of consciousness	• **Mortality:** Delirious patients had significantly higher hospital death rates (23%), compared with demented (4%), depressed (5%), or cognitively intact patients (4%). At 1-year follow-up, delirious patients still had higher death rates than demented patients (46% *vs.* 25%), but not statistically significant.	Analyses do not control for confounders, e.g., illness severity, comorbidity, age, baseline functional status. Relatively small numbers of deaths at 1-year follow-up, with substantial losses to follow-up. Pre-DSM definition of delirium.

Table 8.4 – Continued

Reference	Population	Method for detection of delirium	Delirium outcomes	Comments
Hodkinson 1973[3]	Multicenter study involving newly admitted patients (65 years at 21 geriatric departments, N = 588 (144 (24%) with delirium).	Delirium defined as recent (<2 weeks) mental confusion, with Blessed Mental Test score < 25/34 at admission.	• **Mortality:** Delirious patients had significantly higher rates of hospital mortality (25%), compared with cognitively intact (12.5%) or demented (19%) patients.	Analyses do not control for confounders, e.g, illness severity, comorbidity, age, baseline functional status. Pre-DSM definition of delirium.

*LOS = length of stay; DRG = Medicare Diagnosis Related Group; MMSE = Mini-Mental State Examination; RR = relative risk; CI = confidence interval; DSM = Diagnostic and Statistical Manual of the American Psychiatric Association

The grain of truth contained in this hypothesis, however, is the fact that delirium and dementia are highly inter-related, and the recent evidence outlined above supports some degree of overlap between these syndromes. Moreover, delirium superimposed on dementia may well alter the trajectory of the individual's cognitive and functional decline, resulting in a more rapid course with poorer outcomes. The results of the study by Levkoff et al[64] on a population with a high rate of institutionalization suggests that persons with underlying cognitive impairment may not ever return to their pre-delirium baseline.

2. Delirium may unmask an unrecognized dementia.

This hypothesis is undoubtedly true, and delirium probably does serve an important role in bringing dementia to clinical recognition in some cases. Many previous studies[80-84] have documented that dementia is often unrecognized by clinicians until its advanced stages. Delirium, and its association with acute medical illness, brings the patient for medical care or hospitalization, and thus serves as a vehicle for detection of underlying cognitive dysfunction. Thus, delirium and dementia remain distinct entities, but delirium does serve to bring the dementia to clinical recognition. The relative frequency of this occurrence has not been well defined, and this is an important area for future epidemiologic investigations.

3. Delirium itself leads to chronic cognitive impairment.

The epidemiologic evidence outlined above, including the persistence, duration, and outcome studies, lend support for this hypothesis, but the results are not definitive. The persistence and long-term detrimental effects of delirium are most likely related to the duration, severity, and underlying cause(s) of the delirium. As

Table 8.5 – Prevention of delirium

(1) Improved recognition and diagnosis:
• Aggressive educational and monitoring efforts to alert physicians, nurses, and other health care professional about delirium • Use of simplified diagnostic criteria • Changing health care systems (e.g., quality review criteria) to provide incentives for appropriate recognition and management of delirium
(2) Hospital-based intervention programs:
• Address risk factors for delirium in older persons: - Dehydration - Overuse of sedative-hypnotics and psychoactive medications - Enforced immobilization and use of immobilizing devices (e.g., restraints, bladder catheters)

detailed above, not all of the basic pathophysiologic and etiologic factors associated with delirium will be reversible (such as prolonged hypoxemia and structural neurologic lesions), and it may not always be possible to alter the patients baseline vulnerability or to remove all noxious insults. Thus, on a pathophysiologic level, there is justification that all cases of delirium may not be reversible.

However, to draw definitive conclusions about the long-term detrimental effects of delirium on cognitive function, future work is greatly needed to establish that delirium itself results in permanent structural brain damage. To date, such studies have not been carried out. Prospective, well-controlled, methodologically rigorous studies (which control for baseline cognitive function, and evaluate patients with and without dementia or structural brain abnormalities) with long-term follow-up will be needed to answer this important question. Use of the newer neuroimaging methods, particularly single proton emission computed tomography, positron emission tomography, and functional magnetic resonance imaging, will provide invaluable information in this regard. In addition, sequential studies with neuropsychological and neurophysiological (electroencephalographic) and neurotransmitter testing before, during and after delirium (including before and after drug trials) will help to further elucidate these questions. Finally, long-term pathologic studies of patients with delirium are greatly needed. Studies of this nature would provide definitive information on the long-term effects of delirium on cognitive function.

STRATEGIES FOR PREVENTION OF DELIRIUM

Prevention of delirium must be included in any plan of strategies to prevent cognitive decline in later life. Acute illness and hospitalization often represent pivotal events in the life of older persons, with cognitive and functional decline representing the most feared, yet unfortunately common, outcomes. These outcomes can be avoided with appropriate preventive efforts. An outline of preventive strategies is presented in Table 8.5. The cornerstone to delirium prevention will be aggressive educational and monitoring efforts directed toward physician and nursing staff, in order to heighten their awareness of the importance and prognostic ramifications of delirium in hospitalized elderly patients. Use of simplified diagnostic criteria, such as the Confusion Assessment Method[77] - a shortened tool designed to assist non-psychiatrically trained clinicians with recognition of delirium - provides great assistance to educate clinicians and to use as a tool for improved recognition in high-risk populations. In addition, changing our health care systems, such as instituting quality review criteria, will be needed to provide incentives for appropriate recognition and management of delirium in hospitalized older patients.

Finally, intervention programs in the hospital setting will be of paramount importance for delirium prevention. These programs should be targeted to directly address delirium risk factors in high risk patients. Important risk factors which can be immediately addressed include: dehydration;[5,16,18] overuse of sedative-hypnotics and other psychoactive medications in hospitalized older persons;[16,18,74,86] enforced immobilization, including use of physical restraints or immobilizing devices (e.g. bladder catheters).[1,87] These are areas where hospitals can implement interventions immediately, and see reduced rates of delirium in their older populations.

CONCLUSION

Delirium, a common and potentially devastating problem for hospitalized older persons, has assumed increasing importance as our population ages. In fact, delirium may be the leading complication of hospitalization for older persons,[8] and poses substantial risk for acute cognitive and functional decline. As summarized in this chapter, delirium is highly inter-related with dementia. In particular, delirium may serve as a vehicle to unmask an unrecognized dementia. Furthermore, recent epidemiologic evidence suggests that delirium may be much more persistent than previously believed, and may lead to dementia with irreversible cognitive decline, particularly in patients with some underlying degree of cognitive impairment.

Although the fundamental pathophysiologic mechanisms of delirium remain poorly defined, clearly some mechanisms and etiologic factors may not be reversible. Future studies are greatly needed to define the basic pathophysiologic mechanisms of delirium, and to determine the type and extent of structural damage which results from a delirium. Applying state-of-the-art neuroimaging, neurophysiologic, neuropsychologic, neurobiological, and neuropathologic studies to evaluation of delirium will be particularly important in this regard.

Finally, strategies to prevent cognitive decline in later life must include efforts to prevent delirium in hospitalized older persons. Preventive efforts for delirium should include educational efforts for physicians and nurses to improve recognition and heighten awareness of the problem of delirium; provide incentives for recognition of delirium in the hospital; and establish hospital-based intervention programs to target delirium risk factors, such as dehydration, psychoactive medication use, and immobilization and dehydration. These preventive strategies hold great promise for reducing delirium and its associated morbidity and mortality, and for potential health benefits to the geriatric population at large.

REFERENCES

1. Levkoff SE, Besdine RW, Wetle T. Acute confusional states (Delirium) in the hospitalized elderly. *Ann Rev Gerontol Geriatr* 1986; **6**: 1–26.

2. Rosin AJ, Boyd RV. Complications of illness in geriatric patients in hospital. *J Chron Dis* 1966; **19**: 307–313.

3. Hodkinson HM. Mental impairment in the elderly. *J R Coll Physicians Lond* 1973; **7**: 305–317.

4. Bergman K, Eastham EJ. Psychogeriatric ascertainment and assessment for treatment in an acute medical ward setting. *Age Aging* 1974; **3**: 174–188.

5. Seymour DG, Henschke PJ, Cape RDT, Campbell ACJ. Acute confusional states and dementia in the elderly: the role of dehydration/volume depletion, physical illness and age. *Age Ageing* 1980; **9**: 137–146.

6. Report of the Royal College of Physicians by the College Committee on Geriatrics. Organic mental impairment in the elderly. *J R Coll Physicians Lond* 1981; **15**: 141–167.

7. Chisholm SE, Deniston OL, Ingrisan RM, Barbus AJ. Prevalence of confusion in elderly hospitalized patients. *J Gerontol Nurs* 1982; **8**: 87–96.

8. Gillick MR, Serrell NA, Gillick LS. Adverse consequences of hospitalization in the elderly. *Soc Sci Med* 1982; **16**: 1033–1038.

9. Warshaw GA, Moore JT, Friedman SW *et al.* Functional disability in the hospitalized elderly. *JAMA* 1982; **248**: 847–50.

10. Cavanaugh S. The prevalence of emotional and cognitive dysfunction in a general medical population: Using the MMSE, GHQ, and BDI. *Gen Hosp Psychiat.* 1983; **5**: 15–24.

11. Lipowski ZJ. Transient cognitive disorders (Delirium, acute confusional states) in the elderly. *Am J Psychiat* 1983; **140**: 1429–1436.

12. Lipowski ZJ. Acute confusional states (Delirium) in the elderly. In: Albert ML (ed) *Clinical Neurology of Aging.* Oxford University Press, New York, 1984, pp 279–297.

13. Williams MA, Campbell EB, Raynor WJ, Musholt MA, Mlynarczyk SM, Crane LF. Predictors of acute confusional states in hospitalized elderly patients. *Res Nurse Health.* 1985; **8**: 31–40.

14. Fields SD, MacKenzie CR, Charlson ME, Perry SW. Reversibility of cognitive impairment in medical inpatients. *Arch Intern Med* 1986; **146**: 1593–1596.

15. Cameron DJ, Thomas RI, Mulvihill M, Bronheim H. Delirium: A test of the Diagnostic and Statistical Manual III Criteria on medical inpatients. *J Am Geriatr Soc* 1987; **35**: 1007–1010.

16. Foreman MD. Confusion in the hospitalized elderly: Incidence, onset, and associated factors. *Res Nurse Health* 1989; **12**: 21–29.

17. Rockwood K. Acute confusion in elderly medical patients. *J Am Geriatr Soc* 1989; **37**: 150–154.

18. Francis J, Martin D, Kapoor WN. A prospective study of delirium in hospitalized elderly. *JAMA* 1990; **263**: 1097–1101.

19. Roth M. The natural history of mental disorder in old age. *J Ment Sci* 1955; **101**: 281–303.

20. Kay DWK, Norris V, Post F. Prognosis in psychiatric disorders of the elderly: An attempt to define indicators of early death and early recovery. *J Ment Sci.* 1956; **120**: 129–140.

21. Bedford PD. General medical aspects of confusional states in elderly people. *Br Med J* 1959; 185–8.

22. Guze SB, Cantwell DP. The prognosis in "organic brain" syndromes. *Am J Psychiatr* 1964; **120**: 878–881.

23. Guze SB, Daengsurisri S. Organic brain syndromes: Prognostic significance in general medical patients. *Arch Gen Psychiatr* 1967; **17**: 365–366.

24. Rabins PV, Folstein MF. Delirium and dementia: Diagnostic criteria and fatality rates. *Br J Psychiatr* 1982; **140**: 149–153.

25. Weddington WW. The mortality of delirium: An underappreciated problem? *Psychosomatics* 1982; **23**: 1232–1235.

26. Trzepacz PT, Teague GB, Lipowski ZJ. Delirium and other organic mental disorders in a general hospital. *Gen Hosp Psychiatr* 1985; **7**: 101-106.

27. Black DW, Warrack G, Winokur G. The Iowa record-linkage study II. Excess mortality among patients with organic mental disorders. *Arch Gen Psychiatr* 1985; **42**: 78-81.

28. Fields SD, MacKenzie CR, Charlson ME, Sax FL. Cognitive impairment: Can it predict the course of hospitalized patients? *J Am Geriatr Soc* 1986; **34**: 579-585.

29. Fields SD, MacKenzie CR, Charlson ME, Sax FL. Cognitive impairment: Can it predict the course of hospitalized patients? *J Am Geriatr Soc* 1986; **34**: 579-585.

30. Thomas RI, Cameron DJ, Fahs MC. A prospective study of delirium and prolonged hospital stay: exploratory study. *Arch Gen Psychiatr* 1988; **45**: 937-940.

31. Magaziner J, Simonsick EM, Kashner M, Hebel JR, Kenzora JE. Survival experience of aged hip fracture patients. *Am J Pub Health* 1989; **79**: 274-278.

32. Rockwood K. Delays in the discharge of elderly patients. *J Clin Epidemiol* 1990; **43**: 971-975.

33. Brannstron B, Gustafson Y, Norberg A, Winblad B. ADL performance and dependency on nursing care in patients with hip fractures and acute confusion in a task allocation care system. *Scand J Caring Sci* 1991; **5**: 3-11.

34. Eisdorfer C, Maddox GL. A distinctive role for hospitals in caring for older adults: Issues and options. In: Eisdorfer C, Maddox GL (eds) *The Role of Hospitals in Geriatric Care*. Springer, New York, 1988, pp 1-2.

35. US Bureau of the Census. *Statistical Abstract of the United States 1995*. 115th edn. US Department of Commerce, Washington, DC, 1995, pp114, 128.

36. Francis JF. Delirium in older patients. *J Am Geriatr Soc* 1992; **40**: 829-838.

37. Romano J, Engel GL. Delirium: I. Electroencephalographic data. *Arch Neurol Psychiatr* 1944; **51**: 356-377.

38. Engel GL, Romano J. Delirium: II. Reversibility of the electroencephalogram with experimental procedures. *Arch Neurol Psychiatr* 1944; **51**: 378-392.

39. Brizer DA, Manning DW. Delirium induced by poisoning with anticholinergic agents. *Am J Psychiatr* 1982; **139**: 1343-1344.

40. Itil T, Fink M. Anticholinergic drug-induced delirium: Experimental modification, quantitative EEG and behavioral correlations. *J Nerv Ment Dis* 1966; **143**: 492-507.

41. Blass JP, Gibson GE. Carbohydrates and acetylcholine synthesis: Implications for cognitive disorders. In: Davis KL, Berger PA (eds) *Brain Acetylcholine and Neuropsychiatric Disease*. Plenum Press, New York,1979, pp 215-236.

42. Blass JP, Gibson GE, Duffy TE *et al.* Cholinergic dysfunction: A common denominator in metabolic encephalopathies. In: Pepeu G, Ladinsky H (eds) *Cholinergic Mechanisms*. Plenum Press, New York, 1981, pp 921-928.

43. Mach JR, Dysken MW, Kuskowski M, Richelson E, Holden L, Jilk KM. Serum anticholinergic activity in hospitalized older persons with delirium: A preliminary study. *J Am Geriatr Soc* 1995; **43**: 491-495.

44. Tune LE, Holland A, Folstein MF *et al.* Association of postoperative delirium with raised serum levels of anticholinergic drugs. *Lancet* 1981; **2**: 651-653.

45. Mondimore FM, Damlouji N, Folstein MR *et al.* Post-ECT confusional states associated with elevated anticholinergic levels. *Am J Psychiatr* 1983; **140**: 930-931.

46. Koponen H, Riekkinen PJ. A longitudinal study of cerebrospinal fluid beta-endorphin-like immunoreactivity in delirium: Changes at the acute stage and at one-year follow-up. *Acta Psychiatr Scand* 1990; **82:** 323-326.

47. Koponen H, Reinikainen K, Riekkinen PJ. Cerebrospinal fluid somatostatin in delirium. II Changes at the acute stage and at one-year follow-up. *Psychol Med* 1990; **20:** 510-505.

48. Krueger JM, Walter J, Dinarello CA *et al.* Sleep-promoting effects of endogenous pyrogen (interleukin-1). *Am J Physiol* 1984; **236:** R994-999.

49. Renault PF, Hoofnagle JH, Park Y *et al.* Psychiatric complications of long-term interferon alfa therapy. *Arch Intern Med* 1987; **147:** 1577-1580.

50. Suter CC, Westmoreland BF, Sharbrough FW *et al.* Electroencephalographic abnormalities in interferon encephalopathy: A preliminary report. *Mayo Clin Proc* 1984; **59:** 847-850.

51. Denicoff KD, Rubinow DR, Papa MZ *et al.* The neuropsychiatric effects of treatment with interleukin-2 and lymphokine-activated killer cells. *Ann Intern Med* 1987; **107:** 293-300.

52. van der Mast RC, Fekkes K, Moleman P *et al.* Is postoperative delirium related to reduced plasma tryptophan? *Lancet* 1991; **338:** 851-852.

53. McIntosh TK, Bush HL, Yeston NS *et al.* Beta-endorphin, cortisol and postoperative delirium. A preliminary report. *Psychoneuroendocrinology* 1985; **10:** 303-313.

54. Mizock BA, Sabelli HC, Dubin A *et al.* Septic encephalopathy: Evidence for altered phenylalanine metabolism and comparison with hepatic encephalopathy. *Arch Intern Med* 1990; **150:** 443-449.

55. Lipowski AJ. *Delirium: Acute Confusional States.* Oxford University Press, Oxford, 1990, pp 141-174.

56. Inouye SK. The dilemma of delirium: Clinical and research controversies regarding diagnosis and evaluation of delirium in hospitalized elderly medical patients. *Am J Med* 1994; **97:** 278-288.

57. Koponen H, Hurri L, Stenback U, Mattila E, Soininen H, Riekkinen PJ. Computed tomography findings in delirium. *J Nerv Ment Dis* 1989; **177:** 226-231.

58. Hill CD, Risby MD, Morgan N. Cognitive deficits in delirium: Assessment over time. *Psychopharmacol Bull* 1992; **28:** 401-407.

59. Kramer SI, Reifler BV. Depression, dementia, and reversible dementia. *Clin Geriatr Med* 1992; **8:** 289-297.

60. Draper B. Potentially reversible dementia: A review. *Aust NZ J Psychiatr* 1991, **25:** 506-518.

61. Barry PP, Moskowitz MA. The diagnosis of reversible dementia in the elderly: A critical review *Arch Intern Med* 1988; **148:** 1914-1918.

62. Clarfield AM. The reversible dementia's: Do they reverse? *Ann Intern Med* 1988; **109:** 476-486.

63. Larson EB, Reifler BV, Sumi SM, Canfield CG, Chinn NM. Features of potentially reversible dementia in elderly outpatients. *West J Med* 1986; **145:** 488-492.

64. Levkoff SE, Evans DA, Liptzin B *et al.* Delirium: the occurrence and persistence of symptoms among elderly hospitalized patients. *Arch Intern Med* 1992; **152:** 334-340.

65. Rockwood K. The occurrence and duration of symptoms in elderly patients with delirium. *J Gerontol Med Sci* 1993; **48:** M162-166.

66. Koponen H, Stenback U, Mattila E, Soininen H, Reinikainen K, Riekkinen PJ. Delirium among elderly persons admitted to a psychiatric hospital: Clinical course during the acute stage and one-year follow-up. *Acta Psychiatr Scand* 1989; **79:** 579-585.

67. Koizumi J, Shiraishi H, Ofuku K, Suzuki T. Duration of delirium shortened by the correction of electrolyte imbalance. *Jpn J Psychiatr Neurol* 1988; **42**: 81-88.

68. Sirois F. Delirium: 100 cases. *Can J Psychiatr* 1988; **33**: 375-378.

69. Marcantonio ER, Goldman L, Mangione CM *et al*. A clinical prediction rule for delirium after elective noncardiac surgery. *JAMA* 1994; **271**: 134-139.

70. Pompei P, Foreman M, Rudberg MA, Inouye SK, Braund V, Cassel CK. Delirium in hospitalized older person: Outcomes and predictors. *J Am Geriatr Soc* 1994; **42**: 809-815.

71. Murray AM, Levkoff SE, Wetle TT *et al*. Acute delirium and functional decline in the hospitalized elderly patient. *J Gerontol: Med Sci* 1993; **48**: M181-186.

72. Francis J, Kapoor WN. Prognosis after hospital discharge of older medical patients with delirium. *J Am Geriatr Soc* 1992; **40**: 601-606.

73. Williams-Russo P, Urquhart RN, Sharrock MD, Charlson ME. Post-operative delirium: Predictors and prognosis in elderly orthopedic patients. *J Am Geriatr Soc* 1992; **40**: 759-767.

74. Rogers MP, Liang MH, Daltroy LH, Eaton H, Peteet J, Wright E, Albert M. Delirium after elective orthopedic surgery: Risk factors and natural history. *Int J Psychiatr Med* 1989; **19**: 109-121.

75. Gustafson Y, Berggren D, Brannstron B *et al*. Acute confusional states in elderly patients treated for femoral neck fracture. *J Am Geriatr Soc* 1988; **36**: 525-530.

76. Levkoff SE, Safran C, Cleary PD, Gallop J, Phillips RS. Identification of factors associated with the diagnosis of delirium in elderly hospitalized patients. *J Am Geriatr Soc* 1988; **36**: 1099-1104.

77. Inouye SK, van Dyck CH, Alessi CA, Balkin S, Siegal AP, Horwitz RI. Clarifying confusion: the Confusion Assessment Method; A new method for detection of delirium. *Ann Intern Med* 1990; **113**: 941-948.

78. Albert MS, Levkoff SE, Reilly CH *et al*. The Delirium Symptom Interview: an interview for the detection of delirium symptoms in hospitalized patients. *J Geriatr Psychiatr Neurol* 1992; **5**: 14-21.

79. Gustafson L. Organic Brain Syndrome Scale (OBS-scale). Abstract 128, Second International Congress on Psychogeriatric Medicine, Umea, Sweden, 1985.

80. Barclay LL, Weiss EM, Mattis S, Bond O, Blass JP. Unrecognized cognitive impairment in cardiac rehabilitation patients. *J Am Geriatr Soc* 1988; **36**: 22-28.

81. DePaulo JR, Folstein MF. Psychiatric disturbances in neurological patients: Detection, recognition, and hospital course. *Ann Neuro.* 1978; **4**: 225-228.

82. McCartney JR, Palmateer LM. Assessment of cognitive deficit in geriatric patients: A study of physician behavior. *J Am Geriatr Soc* 1985; **33**: 467-471.

83. O'Connor DW, Pollitt PA, Hyde JB, Brook CPB, Reiss BB, Roth M. Do general practitioners miss dementia in elderly patients? *Br Med J* 1988; **297**: 1107-1110.

84. vonAmmon Cavanaugh S. The prevalence of emotional and cognitive dysfunction in a general medical population: Using the MMSE, GHQ, and BDI. *Gen Hosp Psychiatr* 1983; **5**: 15-24.

85. Trzepacz PT, Baker RW, Greenhouse J. A simple rating scale for delirium. *Psychiatr Res* 1988; **23**:89-97.

86. Schor JD, Levkoff SE, Lipsitz LA *et al*. Risk factors for delirium in hospitalized elderly. *JAMA* 1992; **267**: 827-831.

87. Williams MA, Campbell EB, Raynor WJ, Musholt MA, Mlynarczyk SM, Crane LF. Predictors of acute confusional states in hospitalized elderly patients. *Res Nurse Health* 1985; **8**: 31-40.

9

INTERVENING IN AGE-RELATED COGNITIVE DECLINE IN LATE LIFE

Sherry L. Willis

One of the recurring questions in this book deals with the distinction between normal and cognitive aging. Is there an implicit continuum between age-related, normative cognitive decline and the more profound decrement observed in dementia? To what extent are there distinct or similar processes going on - one leading to slow decline and the other to severe decline? What factors differentiate the older adult who exhibits a small degree of cognitive change but then stabilizes or declines very slowly versus another older adult with a similar early trajectory who becomes demented? These are complex questions that are the focus of extensive research and that will most likely involve answers as complex as the questions themselves.

The focus of this chapter is the factors that differentiate normal age-related intellectual decline and pathological cognitive aging - that is, the considerable plasticity in cognitive functioning exhibited in the nondemented, healthy elderly. Older adults living in the community have shown significant improvement in performance on a number of mental abilities as a result of relatively brief behavioral interventions; training improvement represents the ability to acquire and recall information. Significant training gains have been reported for mental abilities, including various aspects of memory,[1-5] inductive reasoning,[6-8] spatial orientation,[9] and perceptual speed.[10] Training studies have found enhancement on complex cognitive tasks including reading comprehension[11] and driving-related skills.[12,13] Behavioral interventions have also been found to enhance older adults' intellectual self efficacy and their beliefs about control of the cognitive aging process.[14,15]

Research on behavioral cognitive interventions with demented elderly has been much more limited and the evidence not so encouraging. In a study of the effectiveness of visual-imagery training among those with senile dementia, it was found that subjects improved somewhat in tests given immediately after the training, but that the improvements were not maintained in later tests.[16] Research by

Yesavage and colleagues[17,18] indicated that improvement can be accomplished by training only in very mild cases of dementia and has minimal practical impact. Recent work by Camp and colleagues has utilized a behavioral approach known as spaced retrieval in which patients in an adult day care center were presented with pictures and given the name of the individual in the picture. If the name could not be retrieved, it was provided by the trainer. The memory interval was successively increased, and improvement in retention of names was reported.[19] On the other hand, maintenance or generalization of imagery based mnemonic training in dementia has not been demonstrated.[20] In summary, training efforts with demented older adults have required much more intensive and lengthy interventions; the magnitude of training improvement has been less; and there has been little maintenance of training gains. Demented subjects have had little success in learning and utilizing the cognitive stategies or procedural knowledge that are often critical components of the training programs shown effective with nondemented adults. Inability to learn and recall these stategies is a major factor in the lack of maintenance of training effects in demented subjects.

This chapter reviews the major findings from a program of research examining the reversibility of decline in performance in two mental abilities in a sample of healthy nondemented older adults. First, however, there is a discussion of a conceptual framework for studying cognition used in our research. Next, several issues regarding age-related cognitive decline in nondemented elderly are reviewed. Finally the chapter presents data from the cognitive training studies within the Seattle Longitudinal Study. Chapter 2 presents major findings on normative age-related change in adulthood from the Seattle Longitudinal Study and serves as useful background reading for this chapter.

MENTAL ABILITIES AND EVERYDAY COGNITION: A HIERARCHIAL PERSPECTIVE

Instrumental activities for daily living

Loss of the ability to carry out the everyday tasks associated with independent living in society is what many nondemented elderly fear most, even more than dying. Inability to function independently is also a hallmark feature of dementia.[21] Functioning in seven domains of tasks, known as the Instrumental Activities of Daily Living (IADLs)[22,23] are often employed in assessing whether an individual is capable of living independently. The activity domains include financial management, meal preparation and nutrition, telephone usage, shopping for necessities, housekeeping, transportation, and medications. Adequacy on the IADLs involves functioning in multiple spheres, including physical and motoric ability, cognition and social skills. Of primary concern in this chapter are the cognitive demands involved in carrying out instrumental activities of daily living.

Assessment of IADL function has traditionally been measured by self-report of the older adult or a caregiver. In our research, however, we have developed several behavioral measures of IADL performance that focus on the cognitive demands of the task.[24-27] The older adult is shown a 'real life' stimulus material, such as an over-the-counter medication label, a chart of long distance telephone rates, or a mail-order catalog form and asked to solve a problem associated with the information on the stimulus label. For example, the older adult might be asked for the total cost when ordering several items from a mail-order catalog, or asked at what time of day it is least expensive to phone a certain geographical region, based on a chart of rates.

While adequate function on tasks of daily living are the practical 'end point' of concern in the study of cognition for both intact and demented elderly, rarely are such everyday tasks the primary variables assessed.[28,29] In much of the literature on normal age-related change, primary mental abilities derived and measured within the psychometric approach to intelligence have been the key variables studied. For example, in the Seattle Longitudinal Study (Chapter 2), primary mental abilities identified by Thurstone[30] have been the dependent variables of interest. In diagnosis and assessment of dementia, cognitive variables from the clinical and neuropsychological literatures have been used.[31,32] Each of these approaches has unique traditions and assumptions regarding the conceptualization and measurement of cognitive dimensions.

Mental abilities and everyday tasks

The question arises of the association between the basic cognitive abilities and processes studied by researchers of both normal and pathological aging and the complex tasks of daily living that are the outcome criterion of concern. Previously, we have suggested that a hierarchical perspective is useful in conceptualizing these relationships.[8,33-36] The mental abilities and cognitive processes studied by researchers might be conceptualized as the intellectual 'building blocks' that underlie the cognitive demands involved in tasks of daily living. These intellectual building blocks should be conceived as necessary but not sufficient contributors to effective functioning in everyday tasks. As noted previously, performance of these tasks involves physical and social skills as well as cognition. Furthermore, instrumental tasks of daily living are cognitively complex and thus involve a number of the abilities and skills of interest to researchers and clinicians. For example, completing a mail order catalog form may involve verbal ability to read the form, mathematical ability to compute the amount of money to be paid, and inductive reasoning to determine the 'best buy' on a particular item.

Most approaches to the study of cognition consider certain of the abilities or processes examined as more basic or elementary than others. From a developmental perspective these more basic processes may be considered to be manifested earlier in the lifespan and to decline earlier than higher-order or more complex abilities. From a neuropsychological perspective a more direct association between these more basic processes and brain structure may be observed. Within several approaches, processes such as attention, memory span or short-term memory, and perceptual speed are considered more elementary or basic.[37] These basic processes are generally thought to underlie and support the development and maintenance of higher-order abilities, sometimes described as executive functions. These higher-order abilities often involve the manipulation of several pieces of information in order to solve a problem. Cognitive strategies or procedural knowledge is often involved in these higher-order abilities. Manipulating multiple bits of information and reaching a solution to a problem is facilitated by the use of specific cognitive strategies. From a clinical perspective measures such as Trils B or Digit-Symbol Substitution are representative of higher-order abilities or executive function. Within a psychometric approach to intelligence, abilities categorized as fluid or crystallized intelligence represent higher-order function.[38] Fluid abilities involve abstract reasoning such as are involved in inductive reasoning and spatial orientation ability (see Chapter 2). Crystallized abilities are also complex, higher-order abilities but development of these abilities is closely associated with education and other acculturation experiences (e.g. occupation) within society. Verbal ability is an example of a crystalloid intelligence.

In prior research we examined the role of the more basic processes and the higher-order abilities in acccounting for variance in performance on cognitively demanding tasks of daily living as described above.[39] Figure 9.1 shows findings of structural equation modeling of the association between basic and higher-order abilities and a measure of everyday task performance (EPT). The basic and higher-order abilities were assessed 1 year prior to assessment of the EPT.[40] Fluid (Gf) and crystallized (Gc) abilities were the only significant direct predictors of EPT. More basic, lower-order processes, such as memory span and perceptual speed impacted on everyday performance indirectly through their influence on the higher-order fluid and crystallized abilities. The effects of age and education on the EPT were also indirect, mediated by their influence on basic and higher-order cognitive abilities. Self ratings of sensory impairment indirectly influenced EPT through their impact on basic cognitive processes (e.g. perceptual speed). Educational level impacted on crystallized abilities, as would be expected since crystallized abilities such as vocabulary are acquired and maintained through acculturation experiences such as education and the lifelong opportunities afforded by education. The sample studied was healthy older adults of above average education. Health-related factors were marked primarily by self-ratings. In a less healthy sample of older adults and utilizing more direct health measures, a greater influence of health variables on cognitive functioning, particularly on the basic abilities, would be expected.

There is general agreement that the earliest decline in both normal age-related decline and pathological aging occurs with respect to the higher-order executive level abilities, as represented in our model by fluid and crystallized intelligence.[41-43]

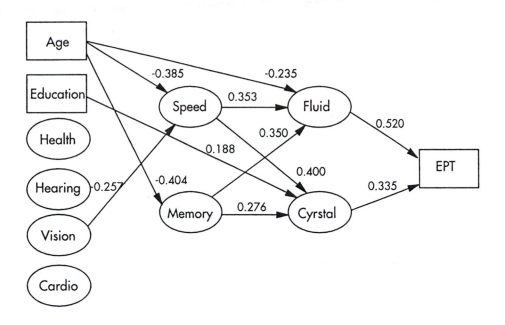

Figure 9.1 – Structural equation model of the association between basic (memory, speed) and high-order (fluid, crystallized) abilities and a measure of everyday problem solving (EPT)

As shown in the model these abilities are most directly related to functioning on independent tasks of daily living. Thus, as preformance on these higher-order abilities declines, some degradation in function on tasks of daily living would be expected. However, as noted in Chapter 2, precipitous decline on even these higher-order abilities is not normative in healthy intact adults, even in old–old age. The proportion of older adults experiencing decline on these abilities increases with age, but very few individuals experience decline on all of the abilities studied within the Seattle Longitudinal Study.[43]

One of the distinguishing features of dementia, compared with age-related changes, is that decline proceeds from these higher-order abilities to more elemental or basic processes. One of the hallmarks of dementia is the dramatic reduction in ability to acquire and recall new information.[21] This deficit is reflected in poor performance on memory span tasks, involving immediate and delayed recall. In contrast, recent longitudinal research on memory span indicated that there is no or relatively little normative age-related decline in memory span until very advanced age.[44-46] Thus, in normal aging many of these basic processes that are hypothesized to underlie and support the higher-order executive skills are relatively intact. Given the differential rate and trajectory decline with respect to higher-order and more basic processes in normal and pathological aging, cognitive interventions for normal and demented elderly would be expected to differ in the target abilities trained. For normal elderly, it is the fluid abilities (e.g. inductive reasoning, spatial orientation, working memory) that show the earliest age-related decline and that have a major direct influence on function in tasks of daily living that would be the logical choice for intervention. In contrast, for many demented subjects these higher-order abilities have declined precipitously by the time of diagnosis and interventions have typically focused on more basic abilities and skills such as short-term memory and name retrieval.

DEFINING AND ASSESSING AGE-RELATED DECLINE

This section reviews several issues related to age-related decline in non-demented elderly. These issues and research findings serve as a basis for our cognitive intervention research that is presented in the third section of this chapter.

Age-related decline and plasticity as intraindividual change

One of the seemingly obvious but often ignored issues is that age-related decline involves changes occurring within a given individual (i.e. intraindividual change). When making decisions regarding whether or not an individual has declined (normal or pathological decline), it is the individual's own prior level of performance that must serve as the criterion. Making inferences regarding whether or not an individual has reliably declined from age-based group norms is problematic, at best, and can result in serious misclassifications. Similarly, judgments regarding whether an intervention has resulted in reversal of prior decline requires comparison with the individual's own performance prior to intervention.

There are wide individual differences in intellectual performance across lifespan and between birth cohorts[43] (see Chapter 2). Older adults of the same age vary considerably in ability performance based on factors such as educational level, occupational experience, gender and health. The significance of educational level as an important variable in making decisions regarding mental status is shown in recent research on the influence of education on performance on clinical measures such as the Mini-Mental Status exam[47-49] and on diagnosis of dementia (see Chapter 4).

Birth cohort membership also contributes significantly to individual differences in ability performance (see Chapter 2). Adults of various cohorts function at different levels on ability measures, even when assessed at the same chronological age. These cohort effects bring into question the use of norms for current young adults as a normative base for decisions regarding decline in current older cohorts, such as is the practice in research on aged-associated memory impairment.[50] Recent findings from cohort-sequential studies indicate significant cohort differences in verbal memory performance.[43] Current older adult cohorts functioned below more recent cohorts when at the same chronological age, suggesting that age differences in performance between young and older adults represent a confound of cohort effects and possible age-related decline.

Selective decline in abilities

Findings from longitudinal research indicate that certain dimensions of mental abilities are likely on average to exhibit earlier decline than other abilities (see Chapter 2). These findings are based on group means and rarely provide an accurate profile of ability change for a given individual. There are wide individual differences in when a given individual begins to decline and on which specific abilities decline is first exhibited. For example, a broad class of psychometric abilities, known as fluid intelligence, exhibits earlier decline, on average, than crystallized abilities, such as verbal ability. Fluid intelligence represents a number of distinct mental abilities, such as inductive reasoning, spatial orientation and figural relations. It is extremely rare for a nondemented individual to exhibit simultaneous decline on all abilities categorized as fluid. Age-related decline in a given individual is very specific with regard to which abilities decline at a particular time. The individual may decline on inductive reasoning, but not on spatial orientation. Given the specificity of ability decline, the clinician or researcher cannot assume that decline on one ability provides conclusive evidence for decline on other abilities – even for other abilities for which research findings at the aggregate (group) level indicate similar decline trajectories. Similarly, the specificity of ability decline implies that cognitive interventions need to be targeted at a particular ability for a given individual, rather than implemented 'en masse' for older adults of a given age or demographic profile.

Variability in ability functioning

One of the most interesting but vexing features of cognitive aging is the variability in function, both within a given individual and between individuals. For many aspects of cognition, variability increases with age. The common reports of older adults of having 'good and bad days' may represent considerable variability in performance within a given individual. Given intraindividual variability in cognitive performance, in both the assessment of intellectual function and in the evaluation of intervention effects, it is important that multiple measures of the phenomenon studied be obtained and that if possible these measures be obtained on more than one occasion. What is of interest in assessment is not performance on a given sure but function on the ability construct underlying a given test score. Obtaining multiple measures is one method for greater reliability in measurement of the phenomenon of interest.[26]

As noted above, the elderly also differ widely among themselves (interindividual differences). Sources of individual difference include age, educational level, occupational experience, social support, health and birth cohort. Variability in a particular dimension of intelligence is likely to increase during the age interval that normative decline is observed. The age at which normative decline is observed indicates that increasing numbers of individuals will decline on a given ability, but some individuals will have declined previously and some will not have declined at all

- hence an increase in variability. For example, an increase in variability with respect to fluid abilities might be expected in the mid 60s when normative decline has been observed. In contrast, increases in variability with respect to verbal ability might not be expected until the 70s, since normative decline is first observed during this decade.

THE SEATTLE LONGITUDINAL TRAINING STUDY

Overview

Most cognitive intervention studies with intact elderly have focused on mental abilities that exhibit early normative patterns of decline, such as those described above as fluid abilities. There has been the assumption that older adults have declined on these abilities and that training improvement reflects partial remediation of prior decline. Longitudinal studies,[51] however, including findings from the Seattle study (see Chapter 2), indicate that these assumptions are too simplistic. There are wide individual differences in the timing of decline and the particular abilities exhibiting decline for a given individual. For individuals experiencing prior decline on the ability trained, training gain would indeed represent remediation of decline, but for individuals experiencing no prior decline, training improvement suggests enhancement beyond prior levels of function. Longitudinal data on prior function on the target abilities to be trained is needed to determine whether training improvement represents remediation or enhancement. The design of the Seattle Longitudinal Study permitted examination of these issues.

The training phase of the Seattle study began in 1984.[7-9,52] Subjects who had participated in the study since 1970 or before and who were 60 years of age or over were identified. Subjects were classified as having declined or not on the two target abilities to be trained, based on their 1970 and 1977 longitudinal data and their 1984 pretest score; 47% had not declined on either of the abilities; 22% had declined on both and 15-16% had declined on just one of the abilities. Although normative longitudinal data indicate that inductive reasoning and spatial orientation exhibit relatively early age-related decline, our classification of subjects according to decline status demonstrates the wide individual differences in patterns of decline.

Participants in the training study were 229 older adults living independently in the community. The mean age of the sample was 72.8 years (range 64-95 years) with a mean of 13.9 years of education (range 6-20). The training study involved a pretest-treatment-posttest design. Subjects who had decline on only one of the abilities (inductive reasoning, spatial orientation) were assigned to training on that ability. Subjects who had declined on both abilities or who had declined in neither ability were randomly assigned to one of the training conditions.

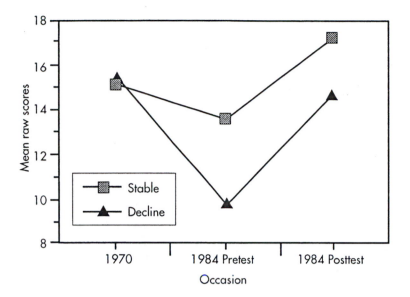

Figure 9.2 – Training gain on the Inductive Reasoning ability.

Given that subjects resided in the greater Seattle metropolitan area, training was conducted in the subjects' homes to maximize participation. Training involved five 1-hour sessions conducted by a trainer. The focus was on facilitating the subject's use of effective cognitive strategies identified in research on inductive reasoning[53,54] and spatial orientation.[55-57] Practice problems and exercises were developed to focus on use of these cognitive strategies. Subjects were taught through modeling, feedback and practice procedures to utilize these strategies in solving problems.

Training improvement

The mean inductive reasoning scores for subjects trained on reasoning are shown in Figure 9.2 for those who had experienced prior decline on reasoning (decline) and those who had not (stable) at three occasions:

a) In 1970, 14 years prior to training;

b) At the 1994 pretest, immediately before training;

c) At the 1984 posttest, following training.[58,59]

A similar patter of effects was shown for spatial orientation ability.[9] In 1970 stable and decline subjects were performing at comparable levels on inductive reasoning. At the 1984 pretest, decline subjects were performing significantly below their 1970 level. Both groups exhibited, on average, significant training improvement. The nature of the training gains, however, was qualitatively different for the two groups. Training gain for the decliners resulted in remediation of performance close to their 1970 score level. For the stable group training resulted in a performance level above their 1970 scores, on average.

Training effects have traditionally presented at the group level, in terms of mean scores. Plasticity, however, is an intraindividual phenomenon – the focus should be in terms of change at the level of the individual.[59] We have examined training effects in terms of intraindividual change as well as average level of change and we have addressed two questions. First, what proportion of stable and decline subjects demonstrated significant training gain from pretest to posttest? Approximately 50% of subjects in each training group showed reliable improvement from pretest to posttest. There was a trend for a greater proportion of decline subjects to exhibit reliable improvement. The second question focuses specifically on those subjects who had experienced prior decline on the ability trained – what proportion of decline subjects showed complete remediation of prior age-related decline? The proportion of decline subjects whose performance at posttest was equal to or greater than their score 14 years previously (1970) was examined. Approximately 40% of decline subjects were performing at posttest at the same or greater level than in 1970, 14 years prior to training.

Individual differences in training effects

While the majority of subjects demonstrated reliable training improvement, not all older adults profited to the same degree from the intervention. One of the most intriguing questions in training research involves identifying characteristics of the person that are associated with responsiveness to training. Our research is beginning to address this issue.

Gender differences

Gender differences in performance on measures of spatial orientation in favor of males have been noted beginning in the early school years.[60,61] Men, on average, perform better on measures of spatial orientation across the lifespan, although there is considerable overlap in the distribution of scores for males and females. While there have been some attempts to enhance spatial orientation ability in childhood and adolescence, there has been almost no intervention in the later part of the lifespan. There is then the question of plasticity in spatial orientation ability in old age. Would cognitive training in old age be effective in reducing the magnitude of the gender difference?

In Figure 9.3 the mean performance is shown for men and women trained on spatial orientation who had experienced prior decline on the ability. Note that over the 14 years prior to training (1970-1984 pretest) men, on average, performed at a higher level than women. Both groups experienced decline in the ability, but the magnitude

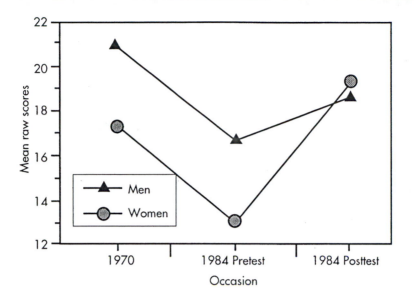

Figure 9.3 – Gender differences in training gain on the spatial Orientation ability.

of the gender difference was fairly constant across the 14 year period. The 1984 posttest data point indicates that the women exhibited greater training gain than men. As a result of gender differences in magnitude in training gain, women at posttest were performing, on average, at a level comparable to that of the men. The gender difference in mean level of performance had been limited as a function of training.

The change scores (1984 posttest minus 1984 pretest) were decomposed into the portion of the change associated with changes in accuracy and that portion representing an increase or decrease in problem solving speed, taking into account changes in number of items attempted both across occasions and across gender.[9] These change scores are represented as bars in Figure 9.4. Each bar represents the total change score with that portion of the total change attributed to change in accuracy versus change in speed. The bars on the left in the figure represent the change over the 14 years prior to training (1984 pretest minus 1970). Whereas for women the portion of the change score associated with a decline in accuracy and speed is fairly equal, a greater portion of the change score for men is associated with a decline in speed.

The bars on the right side of Figure 9.4 show difference scores representing pretest-posttest change. Note that for women the change score on the left and right sides of the figure are roughly equivalent in magnitude. Women regained through training about as much as they had lost as a result of age-related decline. This is not true for men. The pretest-posttest change score (right side) for men in less than the magnitude of the age-related decline (left side).

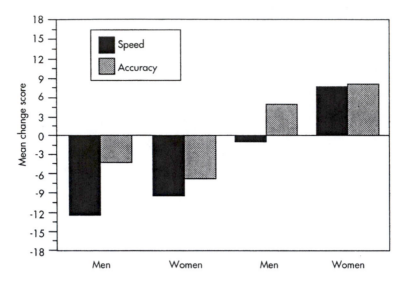

Figure 9.4 – Change of speed and accuracy on the Spatial Orientation ability.

The two change scores (1970-1984 pretest; pretest-posttest) differ for men and women not only in total magnitude of the change, but also qualitatively - in the proportion of the total change attributed to accuracy versus speed. For women, training gain (pretest-posttest) reflected an improvement in both accuracy and speed of performance. Women attempted more items at posttest than at pretest and answered more of these items correctly. The pretest-posttest change score was almost a mirror image of the age-related decline (1970-1984 pretest). Women declined in both speed and accuracy over the 14 years prior to training, but as a result of the intervention they regained what they had lost in terms of both speed and accuracy. Comparison of the two change scores for men present a different picture. Age-related decline for men also involved a loss in speed and accuracy. Training improvement for men, however, represented primarily regaining some of the loss in accuracy; virtually none of the age-related decline associated with speed was remediated as a function of training. Gender differences in training improvement thus reflect not only differences in the magnitude of training gain, but also in the qualitative nature of the improvement associated with the intervention.

Cohort differences

One of the major findings from the Seattle Longitudinal Study has been the significant differences in level of performance when different birth cohorts are compared at the same chronological age[43] (see Chapter 2). Based on the 'American dream', it might be expected that each succeeding cohort would do better than the previous cohort. However, the nature of these cohort effects varies across different mental abilities. For some abilities, such as numerical ability, there are negative cohort trends with recent cohorts performing less well than selected prior cohorts, when compared at the same chronological age. Of particular interest here are the cohort trends for the two fluid abilities that were the target of training. What is the nature of cohort effects for these two abilities? How were these cohort differences affected by cognitive interventions? Both inductive reasoning and spatial orientation show positive cohort trends with recent cohorts performing at a higher level than prior cohorts when compared at the same chronological age. Inductive reasoning exhibits the strongest positive cohort trend of the abilities studied within the Seattle Longitudinal Study. Older adults who have experienced prior age-related decline are, then, at double jeopardy for those abilities, such as inductive reasoning, showing positive cohort trends. When compared to more recent cohorts, the performances of these elderly were lower, on average, due to cohort effects even prior to the onset of age-related decline, which depressed their scores even further.

Figure 9.5 shows the mean scores on inductive reasoning for three birth cohorts trained on that ability at four measurement occasions (1970, 1977, 1984 pretest and 1984 posttest). The three birth cohorts were: the 1903 birth cohorts shown at ages 67, 74 and 81 years; the 1910 birth cohort shown at 60, 67 and 74; and the 1917 birth cohort shown at ages 53, 60 and 67.[59] Significant age-related decline on inductive reasoning occurred for the 1903 and 1910 cohorts (left side of Fig. 9.5) prior to training. The performance of the 1917 cohort was relatively stable over the 1970–

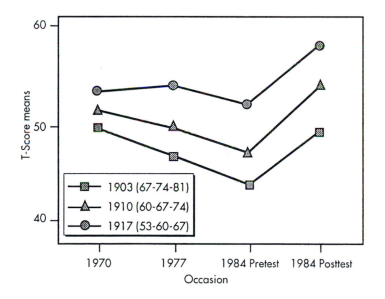

Figure 9.5 – Cohort differences in training gain on the Inductive Reasoning ability

1984 period, since they were middle-aged during most of this interval. Significant training gain occurred for all three cohorts, but there are qualitative differences in the nature of the training improvement for various cohorts. Note that after training the 1910 and 1917 cohorts were performing, on average, at a level above their 1970 base. Thus, for those cohorts in young-old age at the time of training, there was enhancement of performance above prior levels. In contrast, for the 1903 cohort, characterized as the old-old, training represented primarily a partial remediation of prior age-related decline.

Three important findings emerge from comparison of training effects across different cohorts.

1. Significant training effects occurred for all three cohorts, even for the oldest cohort that was in the late 70s and early 80s at the time of training.

2. The nature of the training effect varied with training representing enhancement beyond prior levels for the more recent cohorts, while training effects for the oldest cohort reflected remediation.

3. Age/cohort differences in level of performance are present at all points of measurement, even after training.

Although all three cohorts profited from training, the magnitude of training effects was not sufficient to eliminate cohort differences in level of performance. At advanced ages the lower levels of performance probably represent not only cohort effects but also increasing age-related decline. More intensive training procedures than those employed in this study may be useful when lower performance is a function not only of the increasing probability of age-related decline, but also cohort differences.

Breadth of training effects

One of the most common critiques of cognitive interventions is 'teaching the test' – training improvement is shown only for the specific material that was taught. There is considerable debate over how broad or general training effects should be. The issue of breadth of training transfer is closely linked to the particular perspective or approach to the study of cognition upon which one's research is based. Given that we have taken a psychometric perspective to cognition, our framing of the training transfer question is guided by assumptions of this approach.[59]

Training effects at the latent construct level

Within the psychometric approach, mental abilities are conceptualized as constructs or latent variables. Functioning on a given ability is not directly observable (i.e. latent) but is inferred from the individual's performance on several measures representing the ability construct. Performance on a single measure of an ability represents a confound of variance common to the latent ability construct and variance that is unique to the specific measure. It is the variance that is common across various measures of the ability construct that are of interest. Training effects, then, need to be examined across multiple measures of the same ability construct. Subjects in our research were administered several measures of each ability and factor scores derived as an index of the common variance associated with the latent ability construct.

For each training group, change in factor scores from pretest to posttest were computed for the abilities trained. As predicted, subjects trained on inductive reasoning had significantly higher mean change scores on the inductive reasoning factor. Similarly subjects trained on spatial orientation had significantly higher change scores on spatial orientation. Training enhancement was not limited to improvement on a single test; rather training effects occurred for multiple measures of the ability trained.[52]

Ability-specific effects

A second important issue is whether training effects were specific to the ability trained or whether training resulted in transfer to other abilities that were not trained. For example, did training on spatial orientation ability result in improvement on measures of vocabulary? Since our training procedures focused exclusively on the cognitive strategies that were specific to the ability trained, we predicted that training effects would be limited to measures of the ability trained. It was not expected that teaching older adults strategies specific to spatial orientation would result in improvement on verbal ability. Our predictions were confirmed. Older adults, on average, showed improvement on measures of the ability trained; no training effects occurred for measures that were not the focus of training.

CONCLUSION

One of the major challenges in the study of cognitive aging is understanding the possible distinctions between normal and pathological aging. We have proposed in this chapter that responsiveness to behavioral cognitive interventions, particularly the remediation of prior cognitive decline, may be an important feature differentiating normal aging and dementia.

Prior cognitive intervention research has shown that healthy nondemented older adults profit from behavioral interventions aimed at a number of mental abilities and processes. Virtually all of the intervention research has focused on abilities that show relatively early age-related decline, based on findings of longitudinal studies. Many of these intervention studies have focused on what we describe as higher-order or executive level abilities. Prior developmental research has identified cognitive strategies that facilitate the function of these higher-order abilities. These strategies are typically specific to a particular ability. That is, strategies for enhancing memory differ from strategies for facilitating spatial mental rotation. These cognitive strategies have been employed in training with normal elderly. In contrast to the focus on higher-order processes with intact elderly, the limited intervention research with demented elderly has focused on more basic cognitive processes. These intervention studies indicate that interventions with the demented require more intensive procedures and that the magnitude of training gains is more modest. Training of cognitive strategies has been very difficult. Retention of training improvement is also limited.

The outcome criterion of critical concern in both normal and pathological cognitive aging is the loss of ability to carry out effectively instrumental tasks of daily living. Inability to perform tasks of daily living is associated with loss of independent living in society. Although inability to perform daily acitivities is a critical outcome variable, objective, behavioral measures of the phenomenon are only beginning to emerge. Cognitive abilities and processes employed in research on normal aging and in the assessment and diagnosis of dementia have traditionally focused on more basic forms of cognition, rather than on performance of tasks of daily living. We offer a hierachical perspective on the association between psychometric mental abilities and performance on cognitively demanding tasks of daily living. In this perspective, it is the higher-order mental abilities that are most directly associated with everyday task performance. More basic processes, such as memory span and perceptual speed strongly impact on these more complex abilities, but only indirectly on everyday task performance. We suggest that those higher-order abilities, such as fluid intelligence, which exhibit relatively early age-related decline, are the most salient targets for intervention with normal elderly. Since these higher-order abilities have typically declined precipitously in the demented, the focus of intervention in dementia shifts to more basic abilities.

Cognitive decline in nondemented elderly can be characterized by several featuers. First, it is important to bear in mind that decline is an intraindividual phenomenon. The individual's own prior level of performance is the critical standard for determining whether decline has occurred and the magnitude of decline. Use of age-group comparisons or of younger adult norm groups in determining age-related decline are fraught with problems. Age-related cognitive decline is selective. There are wide individual differences in the particular abilities that show decline for a given individual. Clinicians and researchers cannot assume that decline of a particular ability necessarily indicates decline on related abilities. Given the considerable variability within and across individuals, assessment of cognitive functioning is enhanced when multiple measures of a given ability are used.

Training efforts in the Seattle Longitudinal Study have focused on two mental abilities, inductive reasoning and spatial orientation that within our hierarchiacal perspective would be classified as higher-order fluid abilities. Fluid abilities have been found to predict performance on cognitively demanding tasks of daily living, but to exhibit relatively early age-related decline beginning in the 60s. Since subjects were part of an ongoing longitudinal study it was possible to classify their prior performance on the target abilities as showing decline or no decline. A major question of the research was whether intervention would be effective both with subjects showing prior decline and for subjects with no prior history of decline on the target ability.

Over 50% of subjects showed significant improvement on the ability trained. Of particular note was that after training 40% of subjects showing prior decline were performing at or above their performance level 14 years previously. There were individual differences in responsiveness of subects to training efforts. Two important individual difference variables were gender and birth cohort. With regard to the question of the generalizability of training effects, training enhancement was specific to the ability trained, but not test specific. Subjects showed improvement on multiple measures of the ability trained.

In summary, cognitive research is suggested as a useful paradigm for examining the distinctions between normal and pathological aging. The focus of prior intervention efforts has been on identifying the magnitude of training effects and the individual differences associated with training improvement. Future efforts should give particular attention to issues associated with the lack of responsiveness to training efforts. Failure to profit from intervention efforts may suggest that more intensive procedures are required for certain individuals, such as those of more advanced age/cohorts. Alternatively training procedures may prove to be a useful addition to the existing methodologies for identification of those in the early stages of dementia.

ACKNOWLEDGEMENT

The program of research has been supported since 1963 by various grants from the National Institute of Mental Health and the National Institute of Aging to K. Warner Schaie. It is currently supported by research grant R37 AG08055 from the National Institute of Aging.

REFERENCES

1. Backman L, Mantyla T, Herlitz A. The optimization of episodic remembering in old age. In: Baltes PB, Baltes MM (eds) *Successful Aging: Perspectives from the Behavioural Sciences*. Cambridge University Press, New York, 1990, pp118-163.

2. Kliegl R, Smith J, Baltes PB. Testing the limits and the study of adult age differences in cognitive plasticity of a mnemonic skill. *Dev Psychol* 1989; **25:** 247-256.

3. Stigsdotter A, Backman L. Multifactorial memory training with older adults: How to foster maintenance of improved performance. *Gerontology* 1989; **35:** 260-267.

4. Yesavage J, Lapp D, Sheikh JA. Mnemonics as modified for use by the elderly. In: Poon LW, Rubin D, Wilson B (eds) *Everyday Cognition in Adulthood and Late Life*. Cambridge University Press, Cambridge, 1989.

5. Zarit SH, Cole K, Guider R. Memory training strategies and subjective complaints of memory in the aged. *Gerontologist* 1981; **21**: 158-164.

6. Labouvie-Vief G, Gonda JN. Cognitive strategy training and intellectual performances in the elderly. *J Gerontol* 1976; **31**: 327-332.

7. Schaie KW, Willis SL. Can intellectual decline in the elderly be reversed. *Dev Psychol* 1986; **22**: 223-232.

8. Willis SL, Schaie KW. Cognitive training in the normal elderly. In: Forette F, Christen Y, Boller F (eds). *Plasticite Cerebrale et Stimulation Cognitive (Cerebral Plasticity and Cognitive Stimulation)*. Fondation Nationale de Gerontologie, Paris, 1994, pp. 91-113.

9. Willis SL, Schaie KW. Gender differences in spatial ability in old age: Longitudinal and intervention findings. *Sex Roles* 1988; **18**: 189-203.

10. Hoyer WF, Labouvie G, Baltes PB. Modification of response speed and intellectual performance in the elderly. *Hum Dev* 1973; **16**: 233-242.

11. Meyer BJF, Young CJ, Bartlett BJ. *Memory improved: Enhanced reading comprehension and memory across the life span through strategic text structure*. Erlbaum, Hillsdale, NJ, 1989.

12. Ball KK, Beard BL, Roenker DL, Miller RL, Griggs DS. Age and visual search: Expanding the useful field of view. *J Optical Soc Am* 1988; **5**: 2210-2219.

13. Ball K, Owsley (???Author – initial??), Sloane ME, Roenker DL, Bruni JR. Visual attention problems as predictor of vehicle crashes in older drivers. *Invest Ophthalmol Vis Sci* 1993; **34**: 3110-3123.

14. Dittmann-Kohli F, Lachman ME, Kliegl R, Baltes PB. Effects of cognitive training and testing on intellectual efficacy beliefs in elderly adults. *J Gerontol: Psychol Sci* 1991; **46**: 162-164.

15. Lachman ME, Ziff MA, Spiro A. Maintaining sense of control in later life. In: Abeles R, Gift JC, Ory MG (eds) *Aging and Quality of Life*. Springer, New York, 1994.

16. Zarit SH, Zarit J, Reever K. Memory training or severe memory loss: Effects of senile dementia. *Gerontologist* 1982; **22**: 373-377.

17. Yesavage J. Degree of dementia and improvement with memory training. *Clin Gerontol* 1982, **1**: 77-81.

18. Yesavage JA, Westphal J, Rush L. Senile dementia: Combined pharmacologic and psychologic treatment. *J Am Geriat Soc* 1981; **29**: 164-171.

19. Camp CJ, McKitrick LA. Memory inteventions in Alzheimer's -type dementia populations: Methodological and theoretical issues. In: West RL, Sinnot JD (eds) *Everyday Memory and Aging: Current Research and Methodology*. Springer, New York, 1992, pp. 155-172.

20. Backman L, Josephsson S, Herlitz A, Stigsdotter A, Vitanen M. The generalizability of training gains in dementia: Effects of an imagery-based mnemonic on face-name retention duration. *Psychol Aging* 1991; **6**: 489-492.

21. American Psychiatric Association. *Diagnostic and Statistical Manual of Mental Disorders*, 3rd edn. Revised (DSM-III-R). American Psychiatric Association, Washington, 1987.

22. Fillenbaum GG. Screening the elderly: A brief instrumental activities of daily living measure. *J Am Geriatrics Soc* 1985; **33**: 698-706.

23. Lawton MP, Brody E. Assessment of older people: self maintaining and instrumental acitivities of daily living. *Gerontologist* 1969; **9**: 179-185.

24. Diehl M, Willis SL, Schaie KW. Everday problem solving in older adults: Observational

assessment and cognitive correlates. *Psychol Aging* 1995: **10**: 478-491.

25. Mariske M, Willis SL. Dimensionality of everyday problem solving in older adults. *Psychol Aging* 1995; **10**: 269-283.

26. Willis SL. Assessing everyday competence in the cognitively challenged elderly. In: Smyer MA, Schaie KW, Kapp M (eds) *Older Adults' Decision-Making and the Law.* Springer, New York, 1996, pp 87-126.

27. Willis SL. Everyday cognitive competence in the elderly. Conceptual issues and empirical findings. *Gerontologist,* in press.

28. Loewenstein D, Amigo, Duara F et al. A new scale for the assessment of functional status in Alzheimer's disease and related disorders. *J Gerontol: Psychol Sci* 1989: **44**: 114-121.

29. Vitaliano P, Breen A, Albert M, Russo J, Prinz P. Memory, attention, and functional status in community-residing Alzheimer's type dementia patients and optimally healthy individuals. *J Gerontol* 1984; **39**: 58-64.

30. Thurstone T. *Primary Mental Abilities for Grades 9-12* (rev ed). Science Research Associates, Chicago, 1962.

31. Folstein MF, Folstein Se, McHugh PR. The Mini Mental State Exam: A practical method of grading the cognitive state of patients for the clinician. *J Psychiat Res* 1975; **12**: 189-198.

32. Morris JC, Heyman A, Mohs RC et al. The Consortium to establish a Registry for Alzheimer's Disease (CERAD). I. Clinical and neuropsychological assessment of Alzheimer's disease. *Neurology* 1989; **398**: 1159-1165.

33. Willis SL. Cognitive interventions in the elderly. In Schaie KW (ed) *Annual Review of Gerontology and Geriatrics Vol 7.* Springer, New York, 1987, pp 159-188.

34. Willis SL. Cognition and everyday competency. In: Schaie KW, Lawton MP (eds) *Annual Review of Gerontology and Geriatrics, Vol 11.* Springer, New York, 1991.

35. Willis SL. Everyday problem solving. In: Birren JE, Schaie KW (eds) *Handbook of the Psychology of Aging,* 4th edn. Academic Press, New York, 1996.

36. Willis SL, Schaie KW. Practical intelligence in later life. In: Sternberg R, Wagner R (eds) *Practical Intelligence.* Cambridge University Press, New York, 1986, pp. 236-270.

37. Salthouse TA. *Theoretical Perspectives on Cognitive Aging.* Erlbaum, Hillsdale, NJ, 1991.

38. Cattell RB. *Abilities: Their Structure, Growth and Action.* Houghton Mifflin, Boston, 1971.

39. Willis SL, Jay GM, Diehl M, Marsiske M. Longitudinal change and prediction of everyday task competence in the elderly. *Res Aging* 1992; **14**: 68-91.

40. Marsiske M, Willis SL, Goodwin P, Maier H. Relationships Among Cognitive Processes, Intellectual Abilities and Everyday Task Performance. Paper presented at the Fourth Cognitive Aging Conference, Atlanta, GA, April 1992.

41. Ashford J, Kolm P, Colliver J, Bekian C, Hsu L. Alzheimer patient evaluation and the Mini-Mental State: Item characteristic curve analysis. *J Gerontol: Psychol Sci* 1989; **44**: 139-146.

42. Reisberg B, Ferros S, de Leon MJ, Crook T. The Global Deterioration Scale for assessment of primary degenerative dementia. *Am J Psychiat* 1982; **139(9)**: 1136-1139.

43. Schaie KW. *Intellectual Development in Adulthood: The Seattle Longitudinal Study.* Cambridge University Press, New York, 1996.

44. Craik FIM, Jennings JM. Human memory. In: Craik FIM, Salthouse TA (eds) *Handbook of Aging and Cognition.* Erlbaum, Hillsdale, NJ, 1992.

45. Field D, Schaie KW, Leino V. Continuity in intellectual functioning: The role of self-reported

health. *Psychol Aging* 1988: **3:** 385-392.

46. Hultsch DF, Hertzog C, Small BJ, McDonald-Miszlak L, Dixon RA. Short-term longitudinal change in cognitive performance in later life. *Psychol Aging* 1992; **7:** 571-584.

47. Katzman R. Education and the prevalence of dementia and Alzheimer's disease. *Neurology* 1993; **43:** 13-20.

48. Uhlmann RF, Larson EB. Effect of education on the Mini-Mental State Examination as a screening test for dementia. *J Am Geriat Soc* 1991; **39:** 876-880.

49. Wiederholt WC, Cahn D, Butters N, Salmon D, Kritz-Silverstein, Barrett-Connor E. *J Am Geriat Soc* 1993; **41:** 639-647.

50. Crook TH, Larrabee GJ, Youngjohn JR. Age associated memory impairment: Definition and assessment. In: Agnoli A, Bruno G (eds) *Mental Decline of Elderly People.* CIC Edizioni Internationali, Rome, 1989, pp. 21-28.

51. Palmore EB (ed) Normal Aging. Duke University Press, Durham, NC, 1970.

52. Willis SL, Schaie KW. Training the elderly in the ability factors of spatial orientation and inductive reasoning. *Psychol Aging* 1986; **1:** 239-247.

53. Holzman TG, Pellegrino JW, Glaser R. Cognitive dimensions of numerical rule induction. *J Educ Psychol* 1982; **74:** 360-373.

54. Kotovsky K, Simon H. Empirical tests of a theory of human acquisition of concepts for serial patterns. *Cognitive Psychol* 1973; **4:** 339-424.

57. Kail R, Pellirino J, Carter P. Developmental changes in mental rotation. *J Exp Child Psychol* 1980; **39:** 102-116.

55. Cooper LB, Shepard RN. Chronometric studies of rotation of mental images. In: Chase WG (eds) *Visual Information Processing.* Academic Press, New York, 1973, pp75-96.

56. Egan DE. An analysis of spatial orientation test performance. *Intelligence* 1981; **5:** 85-100.

58. Willis SL. Contributions of cognitive training research to understanding late life potential. In: Perlmutter M (ed) *Late Life Potential.* Gerontological Society of America, Washington, DC, 1990, pp. 25-42.

59. Willis SL. Current issues in cognitive training research. In: Lovelace E (ed). *Aging and Cognition: Mental Processes, Self Awareness and Interventions.* Elsevier, Amsterdam, 1990, pp. 253-280.

60. Linn M, Petersen A. Emergence and characterization of sex differences in spatial ability: A meta-analysis. *Child Dev* 1985; **56:** 1479-1489.

61. McGee M. Human spatial abilities: psychometic studies and environmental, genetic, hormonal and neurological influences. *Psychol Bull* 1979; **86:** 889-917.

10

POLICY AND RESEARCH IMPLICATIONS

Howard Fillit & Robert N. Butler

POLICY IMPLICATIONS: PUTTING CURRENT KNOWLEDGE IN AN HISTORICAL PERSPECTIVE

*I*n 1975, there where only 12 research grants supported by the National Institutes of Health and the Alcohol, Drug Abuse and Mental Health Administration. These grants averaged about $60,000 each and totalled $700,000. There was essentially no public policy (or politics for that matter) that encouraged funding for the study of the dementias. Indeed, among the 11 institutes of the National Institutes of Health that existed at that time, the neurology and mental health institutes were not generously supported, and the National Institute on Aging (NIA) was just forming. Health advocacy groups such as the Multiple Sclerosis Society advocated for various neurological and neuromuscular conditions, but there was no Alzheimer's Disease Association before 1980.

It was former Senator Thomas Eagleton who held the first Congressional hearings on Alzheimer's disease in which families reported the pain and indignity, as well as the financial and personal burdens, brought about by Alzheimer's disease. By 1980, the NIA became the coordinating institute to carry out a major new initiative on Alzheimer's disease at the National Institutes of Health. The neurology, infectious disease, and mental health institutes collaborated with the NIA to establish Alzheimer's disease as a national priority, and it soon became a household word.

Although we know of no conspiracy against the study of the brain, it seems evident that even today members of Congress are not generally aware of the fact that neurological research is on the threshold of remarkable discoveries and should receive fresh resources. The 1990's were designated as the Decade of the Brain. Yet in 1996, there is still only modest funding from the public and private sectors for the diseases of the central nervous system despite growing knowledge of the central nervous system in general and knowledge of the genetics, pathobiology and pathogenesis of Alzehimer's disease and other dementias in particular. These findings alone should give us two powerful incentives to support the Decade of the Brain.

Moreover, attention needs to be diverted toward understanding and preventing the vascular dementias. Hypertension is one of the leading causes of vascular dementia. Efforts to prevent this silent disease had begun to be quite successful in the 1970's. In 1984, the NIA and the National Heart, Lung and Blood Institute inaugurated the Systolic Hypertension in the Elderly Program (SHEP), the results of which confirmed the need for active treatment of isolated systolic hypertension. Wide application of the SHEP findings should help further to reduce stroke and other complications of high blood pressure including dementia.

A different thread of research contributing to our understanding of cognitive decline derives from the fields of gerontology and psychology. Considerable work has been accomplished through longitudinal studies at Duke, the National Institute of Mental Health, and the NIA's Baltimore Longitudinal Study on Aging. The results of these studies have demonstrated that contrary to conventional wisdom, cognitive decline occurs later and is present less frequently than expected in healthy community-residing older persons. But so-called benign senile forgetfulness or age-related memory impairment is still not fully understood. For example, we do not know if this condition (or conditions) eventuates in dementia over time or remains stationary. We do not know if such cognitive decline is an intrinsic part of growing older or reflects a pathophysiological phenomenon, such as atherosclerosis, that may not be fully elucidated but might eventually be preventable. Furthermore, in studying the pathology of cognitive decline and the dementias we often learn about normal behavior, in this instance about the intellectual functions of memory, judgment, orientation, comprehension, and language. Information about these conditions broadens our understanding of central nervous system function in general and resulting human behavior.

It is in this historical context that we comment upon the policy implications of Strategies for Delaying Cognitive Decline. It is imperative that decision-makers recognize the remarkable savings in cost and human dignity, as well as new opportunities for the continuing productive contributions of older persons, that can result from research leading to successful prevention and/or treatment of cognitive decline. The present state of knowledge is sufficient to encourage decision-makers to provide major additional funding to support such studies.

The late Lewis Thomas called Alzheimer's disease the 'Disease of the Century'. As we approach the 21st century, we can see ever growing numbers and proportions of older persons throughout the entire developing as well as developed world. Thomas's powerful phrase will therefore have even greater relevance in the near future. Both the policy and research applications of the work described in this book and elsewhere justify broad expansion of support for research in basic neurobiology and human cognitive aging.

Cognitive decline and cognitive frailty in late life may be neither inevitable nor irreversible.[1,2] With current knowledge, much of what we consider inevitable mental and physical frailty may be reversible. Perhaps one of the best delineated and objectively measurable findings is the decline in processing speed which older people suffer[3] and which affects most cognitive abilities. Physical exercise may have important effects on age-associated cognitive impairment. Aerobic exercise may improve cognition directly by improving processing speed,[4] and indirectly by reducing the risk for cardiovascular and cerebrovascular disease. In addition, from a functional perspective, knowing that processing speed slows with age, we can improve the function of the elderly by, for example, slowing the timing of traffic lights so that older persons can get across streets safely. Finally, cognitive training may also improve cognitive function in the very old.[5,6] Enrichment of the environment, 'titrated' to offer stimuli of appropriate intensity, is likely to enhance quality of life as well as intellectual function for older adults.

More research is needed to understand the mechanisms of age-associated cognitive decline, and the factors which can promote cognitive health in old age. Most research concerning the identification of risk factors for cognitive impairment in old age has focused on risk factors for dementia.[7,8] Limited research has considered decline in executive or higher-order cognitive functions.[6] The few empirical studies that have been conducted have used small convenience or volunteer samples and most have lacked adequate comparison groups. A major impediment to large-scale population based studies is the relative lack of appropriate methodology and instruments to assess a broad range of capacity across multiple cognitive dimensions in a concise manner. Moreover, since change in function over time is the relevant outcome for an individual, studies employing observation periods extended over several years with multiple assessments of varied functions need to be performed. The assessment tools used for these studies must possess good test–retest reliability (controlling for learning and memory) and be sensitive to small changes over time. The measurement of lifestyle and behavioral attributes also requires further refinement to better identify and understand practices that promote maintenance of cognitive function. For example, current methods to assess physical activity and exercise in older persons do not adequately capture the full range of activities performed by older persons and their levels of participation in those activities. Techniques to measure exposure to and participation in cognitively stimulating activities are also lacking.

The capacity to function is used as a criterion for determining the clinical significance of cognitive decline.[9] Most commonly used measures of function for thresholds of dementia generally involve relatively primitive levels of functioning, such as the activities of daily living necessary for basic self care, and the instrumental activities of daily living necessary for management of life and property.[10,11] These latter functional criteria include, for example, the ability to use a telephone, manage one's medications and finances, walk independently, take transportation, and do housekeeping and shopping. Were the goal of old age simply basic independent survival, then these current criteria to determine the clinical significance of age-associated cognitive decline in late life adapted from a disease (dementia) model would be adequate. However, to promote the robust cognitive health in late life, our current notions of 'normal' cognitive aging need to be modified considerably. The 'floor' set by using functional measures which address only the instrumental and basic activities of daily living is too low for these purposes. We need to 'raise the bar' for what we consider the normal developmental curve for cognitive health in late life by incorporating into clinical practice standards regarding the ability to adequately perform 'advanced activities of daily living', which include effective social, occupational and recreational functioning.[12]

In the era of cost-containment and managed care, quality of care and utilization management issues related to diagnosis of age-associated cognitive decline justifiably require careful consideration. There are currently serious problems in distinguishing between age-associated cognitive decline and mild cognitive impairment which represents the early onset of dementia. Screening for age-associated cognitive decline would require significant investments in personnel and time. A diagnosis of age-associated cognitive decline must be linked to strategies for the management and treatment of this problem, which will generate further costs. The cost-effectiveness of screening and management and treatment strategies for age-associated cognitive decline has not been demonstrated. Nevertheless, as Medicare managed care grows at an exponential rate during the coming years, managed care systems can expect increasing numbers of patients visiting physicians and complaining of symptoms consistent with age-associated cognitive decline.

'Preventive geriatrics' will become increasingly important in an era of managed care. Since a small, but significant, number of individuals with age-associated cognitive decline do develop dementia,[13] and since dementia is an enormously costly illness,[14] clinical programs based on current and evolving knowledge to prevent the progression of age-associated cognitive decline to dementia fits well within the agenda of managed care.

Promoting healthy lifestyles with a focus on cognitive health would go far to improve our efforts at promoting productive aging, that is the continuing active participation of older persons in society which allows them to contribute their skills and knowledge through voluntary or paid activities.[15,16] As a society, we can set a standard of robust cognitive health as a goal for late life. Public health measures, such as informational campaigns directed to health care providers and the lay public that promote healthy lifestyles for the specific purpose of maintaining vigorous cognitive health, may positively affect most older persons and help prevent reversible causes of age-associated cognitive impairment. For example, educational programs which communicate existing information about the fact that exercise and control of hypertension can reduce the risk of both age-associated cognitive impairment and the vascular-related dementias, in addition to their well-known effects on heart disease and stroke, may be cost-effective and well received measures for promoting cognitive health in old age and reducing the burden of cognitive impairment on society.[17]

We also need to set clinical practice standards for evaluating and promoting cognitive health in late life. Practical clinical methods for the evaluation of those components of cognitive health critical to productive aging are lacking. Screening measures generally applied to the identification of disease populations[18] are too insensitive for the measurement of cognitive health. Better methods for assessment need to be developed so that an appropriate level of sensitivity for measuring cognitive health can be achieved on a practical basis in the clinician's office. Promoting the concept of late life as a stage of 'adult development' would change current perceptions of inevitable cognitive decline and suggest the potential for continuing cognitive health and growth throughout the life span.[2]

Incorporating these concepts into clinical practice would assist in the early identification of those individuals who are declining at a more rapid rate within the normal range and are 'dropping off' the normal developmental curve. Previous attempts at identifying and evaluating age-associated cognitive impairment have 'medicalized' the problem with terms such as 'benign senescent forgetfulness'.[19] Such approaches do not address the more positive concept of cognitive health. The early identification of individuals with declining cognitive health would facilitate the implementation of interventions aimed at improving their cognitive health or slowing the progression of cognitive decline, such as control of potentially reversible risk factors, and might ultimately reduce the prevalence of dementia.[20,21]

The public health issues associated with cognitive health obviously impact on health policy. While it is well recognized that dementia is a common cause of disability and is extremely costly to society,14 we have little information on the societal and individual costs of impaired cognitive health in the elderly. For example, mild cognitive impairment in the elderly can predispose individuals to be homebound and non-productive, and begin a cycle of social isolation, poor nutrition, and depression, which can ultimately lead to morbid disease complications.[22] Cognitive impairment can also have an enormous impact on the health of caregivers.[23] We need more information on the potential cost-effectiveness of programs which focus on promoting the importance of healthy lifestyles and the control of risk factors as a way of improving cognitive health in old age.

An important and unanswered health policy issue regarding the promotion of cognitive health in the elderly relates to drug development.[24,25] Cognitive enhancers for the treatment of dementia[26] will almost certainly be applied to elderly individuals with 'normal' cognitive decline in the future. A serious issue is the problem of exact criteria for the diagnosis of age-associated memory impairment.[27] Criteria which are too broad may result in huge numbers of elderly individuals being placed on cognitive enhancers, while criteria which are too restrictive may deny effective treatment to some individuals who are truly disturbed by or functionally impaired by age-associated cognitive decline. As in the criteria for the diagnosis of dementia, criteria for determining how age-associated cognitive decline impairs daily function would be useful in evaluating the effectiveness of new drugs. However, scales which are appropriate to higher levels of daily function than those currently employed for the diagnosis of dementia need to be developed which incorporate both the advanced activities of daily living as well as quality of life measures. Studies regarding the impact of cognitive enhancers on age-associated cognitive decline, quality of life and productive aging, including the pharmaco-economic impact, are needed in order to formulate drug development strategies with appropriate and acceptable goals focusing on the promotion of robust cognitive health and function in late life.

CONCLUSION

As the number of individuals living to be very old grows rapidly, the maintenance of cognitive health is becoming increasingly important to individuals and to society.[22,28] Cognitive health is an important component of overall functional health and quality of life. As we approach the end of the 'Decade of the Brain', we should modify our current disease model of cognition in old age and begin to consider the goal of promoting robust cognitive health in late life. As previously recommended by the NIA,[29] a research agenda and a national program for promoting cognitive health in late life needs to be developed and funds from government, private philanthropy, and industry, including managed care companies, need to be committed to implement such programs. As preventive medicine and health maintenance become increasingly important in our health care system, the promotion and maintenance of cognitive health in old age should be a vital and crucial part of health care programs for the elderly.

REFERENCES

1 Schaie KW, Willis SL. Can decline in adult intellectual functioning be reversed? *Develop Psychol* 1986; **22**: 223.

2. Cohen GD. Creativity and aging: relevance to research, practice and policy. *J Geriatr Psychiatr* 1994; **2**: 277.

3. Schaie KW. Perceptual speed in adulthood: cross-sectional and longitudinal studies. *Psychol Aging* 1989; **4**: 443.

4. Spirduso WW. Physical fitness, aging, and psychomotor speed: a review. *J Gerontol* 1980; **35**: 850.

5. Willis SL. Cognitive training and everyday competence. *Ann Rev Geriatr Gerontol* 1987; **7**: 159.

6. Schaie KW. The course of intellectual development. *Gerontologist* 1994; **33**: 580.

7. Heyman A, Wilkinson WE, Stafford JA, Helms MJ, Sigmon AG, Weinberg T. Alzheimer's disease: a study of epidemiologic aspects. *Ann Neurol* 1986; **15**: 335.

8. Mortimer JA. Epidemiology of dementia: cross cultural comparisons. *Adv Neurol* 1990; **51**: 27.

9. American Psychiatric Association Committee on Nomenclature and Statistics. 1994. *Diagnostic and Statistical Manual of Mental Disorders*. American Psychiatric Association, Washington, DC, 1994.

10. Lawton MP, Brody EM. Assessment of older people: self-maintaining and instrumental activity of older daily living. *Gerontologist* 1969; **9**: 179.

11. Katz S, Stroud MW III. Functional assessment in geriatrics. *J Am Geriatr Soc* 1989; **37**: 267.

12. Reuben DB, Laliberte L, Hiris J, Mor V. A hierarchical exercise scale to measure function at the advanced activities of daily living. *J Am Geriatr Soc* 1990; **38**: 855.

13. Hanninen T, Hallikainen M, Koivisto K et al. A followup study of age-associated memory impairment: neuropsychological predictors of dementia. *J Am Geriatr Soc* 1995; **43**: 1007.

14. Ernst RL, Hay JW. The US economic and social costs of Alzheimer's disease revisited. *Am J Pub Health* 1994; **84**: 1261.

15. Glass TA, Seeman TE, Herzog AR, Kahn R, Berkman LF. Change in productive activity in late adulthood: MacArthur studies of successful aging. *J Gerontol* 1995; **50B**: S65.

16. Birren JE. Age, comeptence, creativity and wisdom. In: Butler RN, Gleason HP (eds) *Productive Aging: Enhancing Vitality in Later Life*. Springer, New York, 1985, pp. 29–36.

17. Launer LJ, Masaki K, Petrovitch H, Foley D, Havlik RJ. The association between midlife blood pressure levels and lafe-life cognitive function. *JAMA* 1995; **274**: 1846.

18. Folstein M, Folstein S, McHugh PR. Mini-Mental State: a practical method for grading the cognitive state of patients for the clinician. *J Psychiat Res* 1975; **12**: 189.

19. Kral VA. Sensescent forgetfulness: benign and malignant. *Can Med Assoc J* 1962; **86**: 257.

20. Breitner JCS. Clinial genetics and genetic counseling in Alzheimer's disease. *Ann Intern Med* 1991; **115**: 601.

21. Hachinski VC. Preventable senility: a call for action aginst the vascular dementias. *Lancet* 1992; **340**: 645.

22. Kelman HR, Thomas C, Kennedy GJ, Cheng J. Cognitive impairment an mortality in older community residents. *Am J Public Health* 1994; **84**: 1255.

23. Moritz DJ, Kasl SV, Berkman LF. The health impact of living with a cognitively impaired elderly spouse: depressive symptoms and social functioning. *J Gerontol* 1986; **44**: S17.

24. Rosen TJ. Age-associated memory impairment. *Eur J Cognit Psychol* 1990; **2**: 275.

25. O'Brien JT, Levy R. Age-associated memory impairment. Too broad an entity to justify drug treatment yet. *Br Med J* 1992; **49**: 839.

26. Schneider LS, Tariot PN. Emerging drugs for Alzheimer's. disease: mechanisms of action and prospects for cognitive enhancing medications. *Med Clin N Am* 1994; **78**: 911.

27. Smith G, Ivnik RJ, Peterson RC. Age-associated memory impairment: problems of reliability and concerns for terminology. *Psychol Aging* 1991; **6**: 551.

28. Garfein AJ, Herzog AR. Robust aging among the young-old, old-old, and oldest-old. *J Gerontol* 1995; **50B**: S77.

29. NIA Task Force. 1980. Senility reconsidered: treatment possibilities for mental impairment in the elderly. *JAMA* 1980; **244**: 261.

INDEX

Printed in the United States
51326LVS00001B/353